George Guthrie

Soldier and Pioneer Surgeon

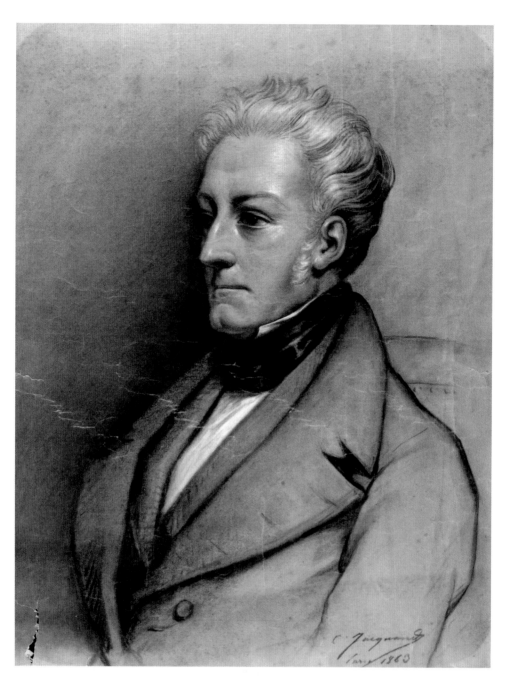

Portrait in chalk of Deputy–Inspector General George James Guthrie 1785–1856 (reproduced with permission from the Wellcome Library, London; Special collection RAMC 952 and 1759/7)

George Guthrie

Soldier and Pioneer Surgeon

Raymond Hurt

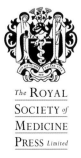

The ROYAL
SOCIETY of
MEDICINE
PRESS Limited

Published by the Royal Society of Medicine Press Ltd
1 Wimpole Street, London W1G 0AE, UK
Tel: +44 (0)20 7290 2921
Fax: +44 (0)20 7290 2929
Email: publishing@rsm.ac.uk
Website: www.rsmpress.co.uk

British Library Cataloguing in Publication Data
A catalogue record for this book is available from the British Library

ISBN 978-1-85315-765-3

Distribution in Europe and Rest of World:

Marston Book Services Ltd
PO Box 269
Abingdon
Oxon OX14 4YN, UK
Tel: +44 (0)1235 465500
Fax: +44 (0)1235 465555
Email: direct.order@marston.co.uk

Distribution in the USA and Canada:

Royal Society of Medicine Press Ltd
c/o BookMasters Inc
30 Amberwood Parkway
Ashland, OH 44805, USA
Tel: +1 800 247 6553/+1 800 266 5564
Fax: +1 419 281 6883
Email: order@bookmasters.com

Distribution in Australia and New Zealand:

Elsevier Australia
30-52 Smidmore Street
Marrickville NSW 2204, Australia
Tel: +61 2 9517 8999
Fax: +61 2 9517 2249
Email: service@elsevier.com.au

Typeset by Saxon Graphics Ltd
Printed in the Netherlands by Alfabase

Contents

Foreword

As a graduate of the Westminster Medical School it is a special delight for me to write this Foreword to the story of one of Westminster Hospital's greatest names. An innovative and esteemed nineteenth century surgeon who has been largely overlooked in standard surgical histories, George James Guthrie has now found his definitive biographer.

Apprenticed at the age of thirteen and a member by examination of the newly formed Royal College of Surgeons at fifteen, Guthrie joined the infantry and began a career as a military surgeon that has few equals. Initially serving in Canada, at the age of twenty-one, in 1808, he was posted to Spain and Portugal to participate in the Peninsular campaign. During the following eight years he gained a staggeringly large surgical experience, treating some twenty thousand wounds. He then served at the battle of Waterloo where, among other notable operations, he performed a successful amputation through the hip, possibly the first ever. As an outcome of this wartime experience he wrote a series of classic textbooks on military surgery in which he detailed many surgical advances. These books were used extensively by army doctors for many years and made him a legend in his own lifetime. After Waterloo he was offered a knighthood which he declined, as not being a rich man he believed that he would be unable to support his wife to the standard required of someone so honoured.

On return to civilian life he at first specialized in ophthalmic surgery founding the Westminster Ophthalmic Hospital in 1816 and later writing three textbooks on eye surgery, especially cataract. Seven years later he was elected to the main Westminster Hospital where he served until he retired. A man ahead of his time, he founded a medical school attached to the hospital which sadly closed after four years and a new and long-lasting medical school had to wait a little longer. However, he was successful in being elected to the council of the Royal College of Surgeons where he rapidly progressed to become President on three separate occasions. During his time as President he successfully argued for reform of an outdated College Charter, attacked nepotism, enabled the end of bodysnatching via the Anatomy Act of 1832, as well as continually pressing the case for improvement in the image and status of army surgeons. He also served as a College examiner for many years.

A forthright man of somewhat brusque and sometimes tactless manner, he was a good linguist, being fluent in Spanish, French and Portuguese, and was also an outstanding lecturer who for more than twenty years gave regular lectures to military personnel without payment.

In this meticulously researched and well illustrated biography, Raymond Hurt brings to life the man and his contributions to surgery in a lively manner enriched by a judicious selection of quotations from Guthrie's own writings. I warmly commend it to all who are interested in the history of surgery.

Sir Barry Jackson

Past President, The Royal College of Surgeons of England

Preface

George Guthrie was a remarkable, and some might think enigmatic, 19th century soldier and surgeon, whose experience during the seven-year Peninsular War led him to revolutionize the treatment of war injuries. He was also a prolific writer, a medical reformer and medical politician, and he was elected President of the Royal College of Surgeons of England three times. Nevertheless he has remained the least documented of his contemporaries – Astley Cooper, Charles Bell, Benjamin Brodie and James McGrigor. It is surprising that a biography has not already been written; he certainly deserves one, as I hope readers will agree. I have done my best to avoid falling into the trap of hagiography, a trap into which it is so easy to fall. Guthrie had his faults, as we all do, but they did not detract from his surgical boldness and skill, his originality of mind or his leadership.

I lost all interest in history at the age of 13 due to poor and uninspiring teaching, but this interest was renewed when I retired and it led to the completion of *The History of Cardiothoracic Surgery from Early Times* in 1996. It was during my research for this history that I became acquainted with George Guthrie and discovered that he had written the first book in the English language devoted entirely to my own speciality, a book which described both medical diseases of the chest and also the treatment of chest injuries. He recorded his experiences in the Peninsular War so vividly and with such meticulous care that they still make fascinating reading. Furthermore, they show that he was a practical and forward-looking surgeon with an overwhelming desire to improve the treatment of battle casualties. This stimulated me to learn more about his achievements and made me realize that the story of his life needed to be recorded for posterity. This, then, is my excuse for this book, which I hope readers will find as interesting to read as I have found it interesting to write.

The book is in two parts – Part 1 is strictly biographical and I have included many of Guthrie's own words in the text (some rather verbose, as was the custom of the time), in the hope that this will reflect some of his character, help to provide 'atmosphere' to the scene and add interest to the narrative. Part 2 describes in some detail each of his many books; battle injuries are described in Chapters 10, 11, 15 and 22 and they provide a vivid insight into the conduct of war in the early 19th century and the type of injury sustained.

With the book in two parts there has inevitably been some repetition of the subject matter, as there is in Guthrie's own writings – many of his thoughts and case reports are described in more than one of his books. For this I offer my apologies, but I believed it was important to make each chapter in Part 2 a complete entity and some slight repetition was impossible to avoid.

   I have delved into the past and endeavoured to include all the available references to Guthrie's life in this biography, though surprisingly these are fewer than would have been expected, and those available are often repetitive. The Royal College of Surgeons of England has virtually no archive material relating to Guthrie, unlike that of his contemporary Sir Astley Cooper. I did, however, obtain considerable information from *Advancing with the Army* (Ackroyd M, Brockliss L, Moss M, Retford K, Stevenson J. Oxford: Oxford University Press, 2006), an exhaustive and in-depth study by five authors in which Guthrie featured prominently and which analysed the social background, army and later civilian careers of army surgeons in the early 19th century. Its senior author had found it frustrating and very surprising that such a prominent 19th century surgeon should have left such a paucity of surviving correspondence which could be consulted.

Raymond Hurt
London 2008

About the author

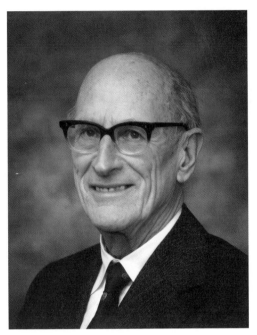

Raymond Hurt FRCS (Eng.), DHMSA graduated from St. Bartholomew's Hospital. After service in West Africa he trained in cardiothoracic surgery at the Brompton Hospital, at St. Bartholomew's Hospital and at Stanford University Hospital in San Francisco before his appointment as consultant cardiothoracic surgeon at the North Middlesex Hospital and later at St. Bartholomew's Hospital. He co-authored *Essentials of Thoracic Surgery* in 1986 and edited the *Management of Oesophageal Carcinoma* in 1989, and his *The History of Cardiothoracic Surgery from Early Times* was published in 1996. He has been Hunterian Professor and an examiner at the Royal College of Surgeons of England and has been President of the History of Medicine Section of the Royal Society of Medicine, the Harvean Society and the Osler Club of London.

Dedicated to the three women in my life

To the memory of my mother, whose guidance during my formative years was so valuable and to whom I owe so much

To the memory of Olivia, with whom I had 38 years of a supremely happy marriage

To Carmen, my newly found soulmate, who has shone a new light into my life, and whose encouragement during the writing of this biography has been so valuable

Acknowledgements

I am particularly grateful to Dr Michael O'Brien for meticulously reading the draft manuscript of Part 1. He made many important and valuable suggestions to clarify and improve the text and reveal certain aspects of Guthrie's life. I thank Mr Harvey White for facilitating the publication of this book – without his help it might never have seen the light of day. I am extremely indebted to Mr M. Crumplin FRCS for his assistance in obtaining information from Halifax, Nova Scotia concerning Guthrie's early army service and marriage, and for providing several images relating to the Peninsular War. I am indebted to Capt. Peter Starling, Army Medical Services Museum, Aldershot, for information concerning Guthrie; to the Worcester Regiment Museum for images of Napoleonic War army uniform; and to Janet Carter of Ancestors Genealogical Services, Birmingham for considerable assistance in obtaining copies of census returns, and marriage and death certificates. Chapter 6 (Presidency of the Royal College of Surgeons of England) has had the approval of Sir David Innes-Williams and Professor Harold Ellis (both past members of Council) and their encouragement has been appreciated. I am indebted to Professor Brockliss of Magdalen College, Oxford for providing extra information from his university's prosopographical database on Napoleonic War medical officers which had not been incorporated in *Advancing with the Army*. I thank Professor J. Richardson for information concerning Rollo Gillespie, whose great-great grandfather was George Guthrie. The illustrations are from several sources – mainly from the Royal College of Surgeons of England, the Royal College of Surgeons of Edinburgh, the Royal Society of Medicine, London and the Wellcome Institute for the History of Medicine, which holds the RAMC archives relative to Guthrie. I am grateful to these institutions for permission to reproduce their images. I am also indebted to The British Library, Churchill-Livingstone, Spellmount Publishing, the National Trust, *The Lancet*, Kew Public Record Office, JM Dent and Sons and Stroud Publishing for permission to reproduce their images.

Hannah Wessely has been the Project Editor for this book and I am most grateful to her for her compulsive attention to detail and for her ready assistance in my requests during its production. Finally the very kind Foreword by Sir Barry Jackson, a former President of the Royal College of Surgeons of England, is greatly appreciated, together with his correction of a historical error in Chapter 6. I have received enormous help from the Royal Society of Medicine, whose library must surely be the most welcome medical library in London, and whose assistant librarian Robert Greenwood directed me to *Advancing with the Army*, a study which I would otherwise not have known. For any omissions of acknowledgement, I apologize.

List of illustrations

Chronology of George Guthrie's life

1785   George Guthrie born on 1st May

1798   Severe accident and treated by Mr Rush, Army Inspector–General

1800   Appointed hospital assistant in June at York Military Hospital in Chelsea

1801   Passed examination for Membership of College of Surgeons of England on 5th February when aged 15

1801   Appointed assistant surgeon in March to 29th Foot Regiment in Winchester

1802   Embarked with regiment for a five-year posting to Canada – mainly based in Halifax, Nova Scotia

1806   Married Margaret Gordon on 7th July, daughter of Walter Patterson, Lieut. Governor of Prince Edward Island, Nova Scotia and widow of Alex Gordon, a surgeon

1808   Embarked with regiment for the seven-year Peninsular campaign in Portugal and Spain

1814   Returned to England, left army on a pension of half pay and joined refresher courses in London

1815   First edition of *Commentaries* published (his major work, which ran to six editions)

1815   Moved to No. 2 Berkeley Street from a small house in Jermyn Street

1815   Recalled to army after battle of Waterloo and served for about five weeks

1816   Guthrie and Dr Forbes founded Westminster Ophthalmic Hospital

1823   Elected assistant surgeon to Westminster Hospital and full surgeon four years later in 1827

1824   Elected to Council of Royal College of Surgeons in London (later of England) aged 39 years

1827   Dispute with Dr Forbes, who challenged Guthrie to a duel

1827   Elected Fellow of the Royal Society

1828   Appointed examiner to the Royal College of Surgeons in London, a position he held until his death

1832   Passing of Anatomy Act

1833   Elected President of the Royal College of Surgeons in London

1834   Guthrie and others tried unsuccessfully to establish a medical school at Westminster Hospital

1835   Purchase of adjacent houses in Berkeley Street, Nos 4 and 5

1841   Re-elected President of the Royal College of Surgeons in London

1843   Resigned from Westminster Hospital to make way for his son Charles

1843   New Charter for College agreed and College became The Royal College of Surgeons of England on 14th September 1843

1844   £12 000 loan to Lord Chandos which was never repaid

1846   Death of Guthrie's wife Margaret from cholera

1848   Death of Guthrie's eldest son Lowry following a stroke

1854   Re-elected President of The Royal College of Surgeons of England for the third time

1856   Married Julia Wilkinson on 26th January

1856   Died on his birthday, 1st May

CHAPTER 1

Family background, medical apprenticeship and war service in Newfoundland

Family background and childhood

George Guthrie was born in London on 1st May 1785. He was the only son of Andrew Guthrie who came from an erudite Scots–Irish family. Andrew had inherited a successful business from a maternal uncle, a retired naval surgeon who had served during the war of the Austrian Succession, and who had developed an improved form of therapeutic medical plaster for 'topical, sedative and astringent application'. The sale of this plaster, together with other surgical materials, had generated a considerable fortune which Andrew subsequently inherited.[1] (Guthrie's father was not a chiropodist, as was incorrectly stated in *The Times* obituary [see Chapter 9, p. 148], though his profession was correct in other obituaries; obituaries have a tendency to inflate the background of their subject.[2])

Guthrie's grandfather, the Rev. Henry Guthry (some branches of the family spelt the name with a *y* and others with *ie*), lived during the reign of Charles I, had published *Memoirs of His Own Times or of Charles I and the Protectorate* and had unfortunately taken the Royal side during the Civil War. He lost everything after the defeat of Charles I and was driven from his home and into poverty. However, by hard work he managed to establish himself again and later became the Bishop of Dunkeld. His cousin, the Rev. James Guthrie, who was an eminent minister of the Church of Scotland, was also an author, but in his writings he had 'denied the royal authority in matters ecclesiastical and was hanged in 1651, his head ornamenting the Nether Bow port in Edinburgh for 27 years'. This was the barbarous custom of the times and the fate of many martyrs who had been charged with sedition. He was the 'great Guthrie' on the martyrs' monument in the Greyfriars Churchyard in Edinburgh. George Guthrie's great grandfather had served under King William of Orange at the Battle of the Boyne 100 years earlier, when the Catholic James II was defeated and which ultimately led to the recent troubles in Ireland.[1]

Guthrie's father had given £10 000 (£656 000 in 2006) to his daughter on her marriage,[3] but sadly most of his fortune was squandered in later life on the services of German quacks, perhaps partly because his marriage had been unhappy due to a nagging and temperamental wife. Guthrie (whom one must assume was younger than his sister) was not so fortunate and received very little on his father's death. The father's marital situation had probably persuaded George Guthrie to leave home early and to seek his own fortune.[4]

From the age of nine Guthrie was educated privately by Monsieur Noel, an emigrant French priest, one of many who had fled from France following the revolution of 1791 and whose reduced financial situation had led him to become an usher in the local school. Guthrie became so fluent in French that in 1814 at Toulouse during the Peninsular War he was told: 'You must be a Frenchman, or the son, at least, of an émigré, if you are an Englishman, which we doubt'.[1]

Medical apprenticeship

At the age of 13 Guthrie had a severe accident and was treated by Mr Rush, then Army Hospital Inspector–General, whom he must have impressed, for this senior army officer soon arranged for Guthrie to have an apprenticeship to Mr Phillips, a surgeon in Pall Mall, and to Dr Hooper, an apothecary to the Marylebone Infirmary, with a view to a future career as an army surgeon. Dr Hooper later became one of the foremost physicians and pathologists in London, and it was to him that Guthrie considered he owed the foundation of his professional reputation. When Dr Hooper retired many years later, he developed diabetes but did not suspect this diagnosis until he consulted his former pupil, who had remained a close friend, and who made the correct diagnosis. Dr Hooper had considered his polyuria ('flow of water' as he described it)[5] to be merely due to his age – a doctor often does not view his own illness dispassionately. He had also developed a prostatic problem and said to Guthrie: 'Mind George, if I am to be cut you must do it'.[6] Guthrie was also apprenticed to William Hunter at the Great Windmill Street School of Anatomy and Medicine (Figure 1.1).

In June 1800, after two years' hard work, Mr Rush considered the young Guthrie to be ready to work as a hospital assistant at York Military Hospital in Chelsea, where he remained for almost

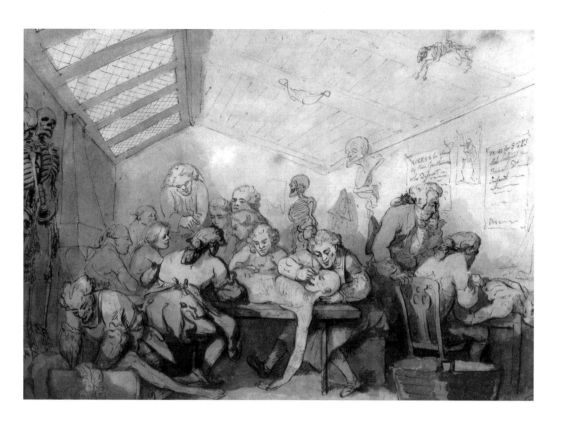

a year. He was frequently dismissed because of his youth and his lack of any formal qualification, but he was always reinstated soon afterwards because of his characteristic tenacity and his repeated approaches to his patron, Mr Rush.

Early in February 1801 the newly appointed Surgeon–General, Thomas Keate, directed that the four hospital assistants who had not been examined and approved by the College of Surgeons be dismissed. Guthrie had been acting throughout the winter as prosector (an assistant known as a 'deputy grinder') to Mr Carpue, the staff surgeon and anatomy teacher at the hospital, and Guthrie considered himself to be at least as knowledgeable as those he had been instructing and who had passed their examination; it was therefore improper for him to be dismissed only on account of his age and lack of qualifications. He did not appeal to Mr Rush but boldly put his name down for the examination on the day that Thomas Keate had made the new regulation. Two days later on 5th February 1801, he successfully passed the examination for membership at the age of 15 (ironically having been examined by Keate himself). The College did not make a minimum age a necessary requirement until a year later.[5]

Figure 1.1 *The Great Windmill Street School of Anatomy – an anatomy lesson in the early 19th century (reproduced with permission from the Royal College of Surgeons of England, London)*

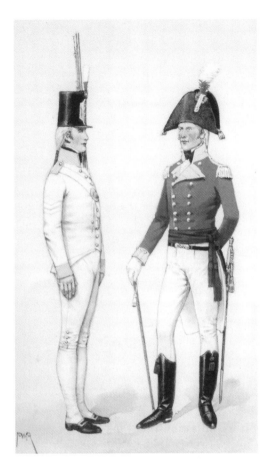

Enrolment in the army

In March 1801, and by concealing his true age, Guthrie was appointed at the age of 15 years to be assistant surgeon (Figure 1.2) to the 29th Foot Regiment in Winchester, again on the recommendation of Mr Rush to the regiment's senior officer Lieut. Colonel Byng, later Lord Strafford, who himself was only 22.

The regiment's full surgeon was much more interested in literature than in his surgical duties and very soon Guthrie was promoted to be sole medical officer in charge of the regiment. It was universally acknowledged that 'there was no regiment that was better commanded or better doctored'.[5] The following year (1802) the regiment embarked for a five-year posting to Canada in order to protect British interests in the New World from American and French aspirations. In 1806, at the age of 21, Guthrie was promoted to be full surgeon. A few years later, when the regiment had returned to England, Guthrie was presented with four silver-covered dishes bearing an inscription expressive of the warm regard they entertained for him.[5]

Figure 1.2 *Left, A private in drill order. Right, an officer of the 29th Foot Regiment (reproduced with permission from Worcestershire Regiment Museum, Worcester)*

The 29th Foot Regiment had established a good relationship with the people of Halifax during its deployment in the New World – first in 1749 to spend a year 'clearing and marking out the site for the future town of Halifax', then 15 years later in 1765 for three years and again in 1802.[6] The town presented the regiment with a silver cup as a 'small tribute to the esteem in which they were held' and their 'sincere regret at the departure of a body of men whose exemplary conduct has excited our respect and admiration'.[6]

Very little is known about Guthrie's time in Canada, though it would appear that he was not involved in treating any battle casualties. On 7th July 1806, when aged 21 years, Guthrie married Margaret Gordon, the 25-year-old daughter of Walter Patterson, the Lieutenant–Governor of Prince Edward Island in Halifax, Nova Scotia,[7] and the widow of a surgeon, Alex Gordon[8] (Figure 1.3).

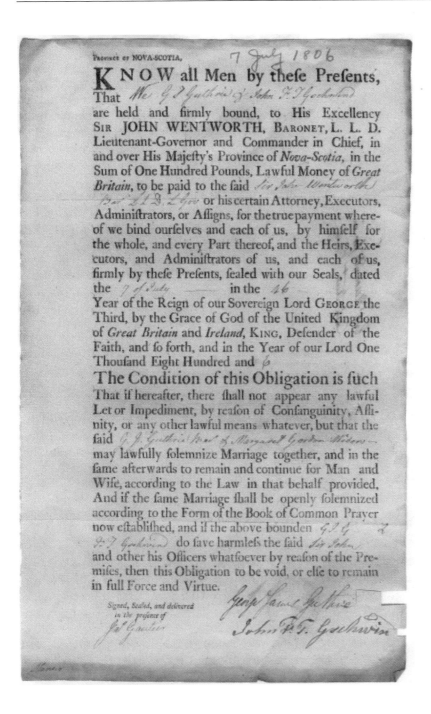

Figure 1.3 *Marriage certificate of Guthrie dated 7th July 1806, for which the fee in Nova Scotia was a surprising £100 (£6560 in 2006). The ink writing has faded over the years but the names of George Guthrie and Margaret Gordon are clearly visible in the original image (reproduced with permission from Halifax Citadel National Historic Site of Canada, Halifax and courtesy of M. Crumplin FRCS)*

The story of Ned – a disobedient soldier[9]

In the 18th and 19th centuries the British army had always had a problem with persistent disobedience and it was thought that to dismiss a man 'upon whom neither precept, prayers nor punishment had any effect' was inappropriate. These men were punished by lashing. Such a one was Ned, who, in the past, had had about 15 000 lashes (so it was said). Nevertheless, he was 'a grenadier of the first order of man, a fellow of the kindest heart, an excellent soldier, but he could not resist rum'. In Newfoundland, in summer or winter, 'for heat or cold were nothing to him', he would swim across Halifax harbour and return with 'as many bladders of rum tied round his neck as he could get money to buy. Of course, everybody got drunk and poor Needham [Ned] was detected and flogged. He never disputed the justice of the sentence'. Guthrie had to witness these floggings on many occasions but he did not approve of the practice of flogging in the army and considered that this punishment was inappropriate and had no real deterrent effect. He thought that 'no man should receive more than two dozen lashes, and that on his bum, in the way schoolboys sometimes get it'. He was not 'aware of any benefit being derived from it. A brand is not affixed to a felon, and it should not be to a soldier'.

Poor Ned 'died in the element he had so often braved with impunity. He was carried off the forecastle of a transport by a heavy sea in the Bay of Biscay, and was long seen buffeting the sea in vain and without hope or prospect of relief. He was the *beau ideal* of a grenadier' (the crack troops of the army).

Knowledge of navigation and seamanship[1,10]

On the return voyage to England in 1807, Guthrie's knowledge of navigation, learned as a boy from his tutor the French priest, stood him in good stead. His troopship had been sailing before the wind up the English Channel during the night and the following morning had to shorten sail due to a sea mist. The captain declared that they were at least 15 miles off the Isle of Wight. Guthrie, however, had been keeping his own reckoning of the ship's position and thought they were less than two miles from shore. Believing he was correct, he went forward to the ship's bow and, peering under the haze, saw land ahead and the buoys marking the passage to Spithead, all this to the amazement of the crew who had previously jeered at the doctor for his outspokenness. 'The sun broke out, the ship changed course, and a fisherman hailed "St Catherines Bay – if you had not gone about you would have been ashore in five minutes".' The captain wished to drop anchor and request a pilot but Guthrie took command and piloted the ship himself to her anchorage at Spithead. He was just 22 years old. Guthrie had said:

> The course was quite clear on the chart; they could now see the buoys, the wind was gentle and there was nothing to prevent their making the port and their way to Spithead, which they did safely to the great amazement of all aboard, at the captain being beat by the doctor, who actually worked the ship to her anchorage.[1]

When the other officers jeered at the captain for having been beaten by the doctor, he replied, shaking his head: 'It is true enough, gentlemen, but it all comes of doctoring, which he believed was something like magic and taught everything'.

Guthrie's seamanship also came to the fore the following year when his regiment was again sent overseas and his transport ship, the *Dominica*, was in the Bay of Gibraltar. The fleet had been beset by storms in the Bay of Biscay; part of the fleet had been driven back to Portsmouth and the remainder eventually reached Gibraltar where they remained at anchor for several days. One night Guthrie was awakened by an unusual motion of the ship; he went up on deck to investigate and noticed that the Rock of Gibraltar appeared in the gloom to be further away than it should have been and that the ship was not swinging on its anchor, head to wind. The ship was clearly adrift.

> On going forward he saw that the anchor was apeak, the cable being nearly up and down and Algesiras was so much nearer than Gibraltar that no doubt remained of their arriving there in less than another hour if their situation had not been discovered. The watch was asleep but they were soon roused as well as all the soldiery; every one was sent to his post and the anchor was got up with as little noise as possible. The ship was now under the batteries of the Spanish and as sail was made upon her they opened fire with some 42-pounder shot, one of which struck the roundhouse on the quarter deck, the others falling short or going over. The wind being easterly the ship had to stretch out into the straits before she could tack to recover her anchorage. This brought her under Cabrita point, the batteries of which also opened upon her, fortunately without doing mischief.[1]

Four hundred men (soldiers and crew) had been saved from death or capture by the Spaniards, who at that time were the enemy, even before they had reached the intended theatre of war.

A further nautical episode demonstrates the problems associated with an overseas expedition in the 19th century.[10] The convoy sailed west from Portsmouth in December 1808 under sealed orders (only to be opened after departure) but there was confusion over their destination, as Guthrie so vividly describes:

> [*We sailed in a gale*] against which we contended in vain. The men-of-war made a signal which we afterwards discovered to be that for the first rendezvous, viz. Falmouth; but the instructions of the master of the transport had it not. The flag was there but the agent had not taken the trouble to have it painted of the regular chequered colour, and this was the case with others, so that we did not know it when we saw it. After 10 days more contention against the elements and accompanied only by one other vessel, we bore up of our own accord for Portsmouth. This misfortune would have been put down to the elements, or anything else, rather than to the negligence of the agent of transports. He had not, I suppose, any yellow paint and could not take the trouble to write against the plain flag that its colour was chequered yellow and blue.[10]

On the way they had met a pirate vessel which 'ran under our stern but, finding us full of men, did not like to meddle with us or we should have found our way to France'. Guthrie also complained that the transports, though maintained at great expense, were often 'commanded by men who were oftentimes quite incompetent; and the loss of ships and lives which frequently occurred' has usually been attributed to 'unavoidable accident, when I have little doubt they really arose from extreme ignorance or negligence'.

Guthrie describes another episode which occurred on his last turn in a transport from Lisbon to Santander. They arrived in the evening and:

> Lay to, with a good fine breeze on shore; the tiller lashed a lee, and the mate and one sailor to keep watch. At midnight I looked out of my port hole and saw the ship was making way fast and approaching the shore, and there was a very odd noise from time to time on deck, as if the tiller was wagging about at its own pleasure. Thither I repaired

forthwith and found this to be the case. The tiller had got loose, the mate and sailors were asleep and the vessel was fast going into Santander, under the guns of which we should have been in another hour.[10]

References

1. Biographical sketch. *Lancet* 1850; **1**: 726.

2. Ackroyd M, Brockliss L, Moss M, Retford K, Stevenson J. *Advancing with the Army.* Oxford: Oxford University Press, 2006, p. 66.

3. Obituary. *Gentleman's Magazine* 1856; June: 649–50.

4. Obituary. *Lancet* 1856; **1**: 519–20.

5. Op. cit. ref. 1, p. 729.

6. Information from Walls M, Mainland NS Field Unit, Parks Canada, PO Box 9080, Station A, Halifax NS. B3K 5M7.

7. Crumplin MH. Wellington's surgeon. *Military Illustrated* 2006; **220**: 48–55.

8. Everard H. *Officers Services 29th Foot Regiment 1694–1891.* Worcester: Littlebury, 1891.

9. Guthrie GJ. *Compound Fractures of the Extremities.* London: Churchill, 1838, p. 3.

10. Op. cit. ref. 9, pp. 24–5.

Chapter 2

War service in Portugal and Spain

The situation of a military surgeon is more important than that of any other. While yet a young man he has the safety of thousands committed to him in the most perilous situations, in unhealthy climates and in the midst of danger. He is to act alone and unassisted, in cases where decision and perfect knowledge are required; in wounds of the most desperate nature, more various than can be imagined; his duties are difficult at all times, are often performed amidst the hurry, confusion, cries and horrors of battle. It is to him that his fellow soldiers look up to at the moment of distress. He has no one to consult with in the moment in which the lives of numbers are determined. He has no support but the remembrance of faithful studies, and his inward consciousness of knowledge; nor anything to encourage him except his own honest principles and good feeling.

(John Bell [1794] – a distinguished Edinburgh surgeon and elder brother of the better known Sir Charles Bell)[1]

The Peninsular campaign

The Peninsular campaign was almost the final episode in the French Revolutionary Wars, usually called the Napoleonic Wars and which could also be described as the First World War, for they had involved the West Indies, Egypt, Spain, Portugal, Russia and finally Belgium. For many years Napoleon had realized that the true enemy of France was England and had therefore occupied Portugal and Spain in the hope of closing Lisbon and other ports to English shipping and thus limiting the ability of England to benefit from their commercial interests in the Far East. By 1806–7 Britain had decided to assist Spain and Portugal in driving the French from the Iberian Peninsula.

The Napoleonic Wars lasted on and off for 25 years, with only short intervals for each side to regroup before the next battle, and during this time major political changes, together with economic and social reforms of momentous impact, had occurred; Spain, Portugal and Russia had changed sides twice during this time.

It has been said that the sword and the scalpel, the military and the medical professions, are closely associated with each other, and, as so often had occurred in time of war, many remarkable surgical advances were made to deal with battle casualties, advances which could readily be transferred to peacetime use. In the early 19th century these advances were led by Baron Larrey and Pierre Percy on the French side and by George Guthrie, who is much less well known but equally eminent, together with Hennen, on the English side.

Guthrie was described in an 11-page biographical sketch in *The Lancet*,[2] somewhat overenthusiastically, as the greatest surgeon in Europe. Nevertheless, he has remained the least documented of that generation of surgeons, unlike Larrey or his English contemporaries Astley Cooper (1768–1841), Abernethy (1764–1831), Charles Bell (1774–1842) and Benjamin Brodie (1783–1862), and Guthrie's military administrative colleague James McGrigor (1771–1858).

Surgical experience in the Peninsular War

It was in Spain and Portugal that Guthrie gained the vast experience of war surgery that formed the basis for his future surgical reputation, his lectures and his seven books on war injuries. Guthrie's early army career had to contend with the reputation of John Hunter (1728–1793), who had been the most famous anatomist and surgeon of the 18th century. His opinions were still considered to be valid at the time of the Peninsular War. But these had rested almost entirely on his civilian experience; his only *active* army experience had been a few weeks at Belle-Île off the Brittany coast. Many of Hunter's opinions for the treatment of battle casualties could no longer be accepted and Guthrie's own opinions, when a young army surgeon in his 20s, were:

> In direct opposition to those of the great John Hunter and his immediate successors. It was the mouse against the mountain. I had every surgeon in that army against me, except those who served under me, and everyone throughout Europe. My papers were read and even referred to by writers. The cases related were, however, considered to be exceptions.[3]

During the whole of the Spanish campaign Guthrie acted as a soldier as well as a surgeon. He insisted on strict discipline and hygiene in his troops, and this greatly reduced the mortality amongst his patients, exemplified by the fact that after one battle the corps under his care, 'with an equal number of men and of sick, had only a line of graves half as long as that of the other two'.[4] This was achieved 'by discipline, not physic – prevention rather than cure'. In the first book Guthrie wrote after his return from the Peninsular campaign, he noted that:

> Young men sent out from England to the Peninsula, incapable of performing any military surgery, become able operators in a short time, from the practical lessons inculcated in our dissecting rooms, in our hospitals and on the field of battle.[5]

Embarkation for Spain

In 1808, soon after his return to England from Canada, Guthrie embarked with his regiment in the transport *Dominica* for the seven-year Peninsular campaign. The regiment's commander was the Hon. G. Lake (who was subsequently killed at Roliça, an event recounted in Chapter 3, p. 33), under the expedition's commander General Spencer.[2] He landed at Puerto de Sante Maria **[1]** on the opposite side of the bay to Cadiz (Figure 2.1). The mission of the expedition was to capture the naval base at Ceuta in Spanish Morocco. It was during this time that the rebellion of the Spaniards against French domination occurred, the mission was aborted and, until new orders were received from England, it was opportune for Guthrie to acquire a working knowledge of Spanish, as Spain had now become an ally.

Battles of Roliça and Vimeiro – 17th and 21st August 1808

In August 1808 the English army landed in Mondego Bay **[2]** (Figure 2.1) under the command of Arthur Wellesley (the future Lord Wellington), having been joined by General Spencer's contingent of 5000 men from Cadiz **[1]**, where they had been lying in transports awaiting their new orders. A total of 15 000 troops advanced south towards Lisbon 80 miles away. No arrangements had been made for the sick or wounded. Guthrie was therefore ordered by Colonel Lake to purchase a mule to carry the instruments and medicines. Guthrie wrote:

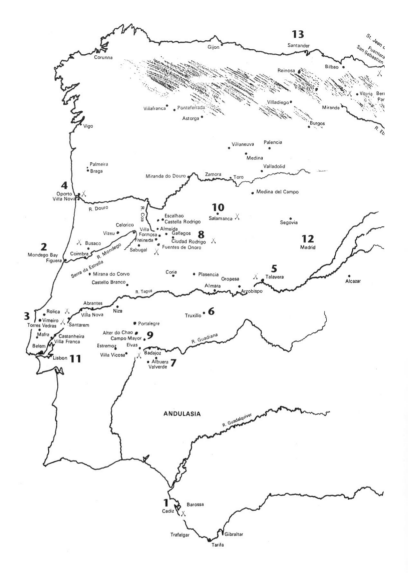

Figure 2.1 *Map of the*
Peninsular campaign.
1. Cadiz, 2. Mondego Bay,
3. Roliça and Vimeiro,
4. Oporto, 5. Talavera,
6. Truxillo, 7. Albuhera,
8. Ciudad Rodrigo,
9. Badajoz, 10. Salamanca,
11.Lisbon, 12. Madrid,
13. Santander

I had two one-handed men attached to me whose hands I had cut off after maiming themselves in America. These fellows could saddle a horse or a mule as quickly and as well as if their hands had not been amputated. They took care of the jackass that carried the physics and surgical stores in a biscuit bag which I begged from the master of the transport, there being nothing else to be had; and thus the regiment set off to take Lisbon.[6]

Almost immediately on 17th August the battle of Roliça **[3]** took place. The main part of this battle involved the 9th and

29th Regiments, the injured of which were all under Guthrie's care as there was no senior regimental surgeon in the field and there was no general hospital ashore. 'His task took three days of unending toil'.[7] The wounded were evacuated to the hospital ship *Enterprise* which had been used for the reception of the sick during the advance. This was Guthrie's first battle experience and he noted that the 200 soldiers wounded whilst storming the high ground 'were all known to me by name or person, and the difference of expression in begging for assistance or expressing their sense of suffering, will never be obliterated from my memory'.[8]

From a mistaken sense of duty, Guthrie had unwisely:

Marched with the regiment towards the enemy, who reserved their fire until the troops actually met, and I saw and heard the first gunshot wound received from an enemy that I dressed. It was on the shoulder, and the soldier described it as a severe numbing blow depriving him momentarily of the use of his arm, and followed by a severer pain.[9]

Only four days later the decisive battle of Vimeiro **[3]** took place, again involving heavy casualties and during which Guthrie was wounded in both legs by a musket ball, 'which fortunately only grazed one and bruised the other'.[9] Both battles were won; the latter is commemorated by a monument (Figure 2.2); they were the first successful British land opposition to Napoleon. Guthrie accompanied the injured (both English and French) to the coast where they were all assembled in a church which was used as a temporary hospital. The scene was described by one of Guthrie's medical colleagues: 'On entering the churchyard my attention was arrested by very unpleasant objects – one, a large wooden dish filled with hands that had just been amputated, another a heap of legs placed opposite'.[7] The wounded were then transported to hospital ships to be later admitted to a hospital in Oporto **[4]**, further north.

Later that month the scandalous Convention of Cintra was signed by which it was agreed that all French troops should return to France with

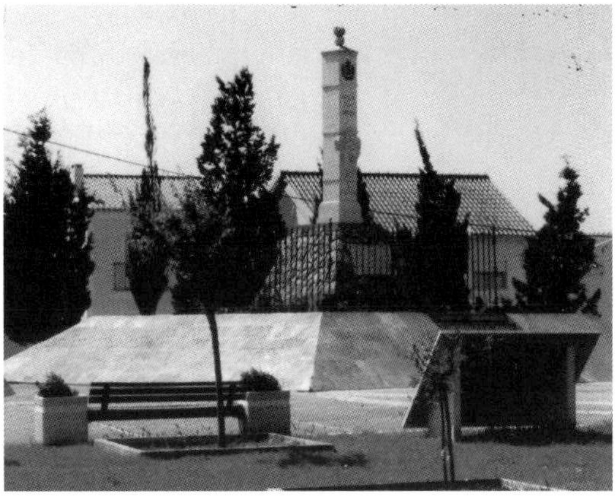

Figure 2.2 *Monument to the battle of Vimeiro (courtesy of M. Crumplin FRCS)*

their booty and equipment in British ships. The Peninsular War became temporarily confined to Spain.

Guthrie was then transferred to Lisbon **[11]** where he not only dealt with the many casualties after the Roliça battle but was also involved in much administrative work which should have been undertaken by non-medical officers.[7] Guthrie had also taken the opportunity to learn Portuguese, which he became able to speak fluently, and this subsequently led to him and his horse being transported by boat across the river Douro into Oporto prior to its capture. He was one of the first English officers to cross and this almost cost him his life. The French had fled the town so quickly that their baggage had partially blocked the town's streets and had been plundered by the townspeople and also some of the soldiers. In the ensuing confusion Guthrie had become separated from his troops and became attached to the 17th Portuguese Regiment which had also rapidly crossed the river, and they offered to show him the road that the English had taken. This brought him under the brow of a hill immediately behind the retreating French. Sir John Sherbrooke, in command of an English regiment, mistook the Portuguese regiment for a retreating French regiment and ordered his own men to present arms preparatory to firing into a supposed enemy. Guthrie quickly realized the danger of the situation and, to prevent an impending catastrophe, tore open the blue greatcoat which covered his red one and held it open. Just as they were about to fire, the whole English regiment called out 'the doctor and the Portuguese' and the impending calamity of 'friendly fire' was prevented.[11] (Guthrie's more detailed personal account of this episode is given in Chapter 3, p. 41.)

Soon after this momentous event, Guthrie came upon an enemy cannon stuck in a nearby lane and, being the only mounted officer present, with typical impetuosity rode down towards it. The driver of the gun dismounted and ran away on foot. However, what to do with the gun? Having captured it single-handed, he cut the traces of the foremost mule with his sword to render the cannon immobile. He brought this foremost mule ('a very fine one') off as a trophy and then sent a sergeant and a file of men to take charge of the gun until he could report its capture to Sir John Sherbrooke, 'who was mightily amused at the doctor's capturing a gun by himself'.[11]

Battle of Talavera – 27th–28th July 1809

Following the successful battle of Talavera **[5]**, it had taken 48 hours to bring in all the wounded, both English and French. Guthrie was promoted to staff surgeon and supervised the treatment of 6000 British casualties. This battle was described as being 'the hardest fought battle of modern times and each party engaged had lost a quarter of its numbers. The town of Talavera became crowded with wounded and those of the 29th, through the activity and energy of Dr Guthrie, were soon lodged'.[6] The Deputy Inspector of Hospitals, Dr Ferguson, was in bed with dysentery and Guthrie therefore undertook the overall medical administration of the whole allied army. This he found difficult because of lack of central coordination, lack of medical stores and too few medical officers, problems which persisted until the arrival of James McGrigor (Figure 2.3) in 1812 as a more efficient replacement for Dr Franck, the Inspector–General of Hospitals.

The lack of central coordination had become acute after the battle of Talavera and Guthrie was so incensed by this desperate situation that he wrote a personal letter to Dr Ferguson, laying the blame entirely on Dr Franck and his assistant Dr Taggart. They had both arrived at Talavera the day before and had found that Dr Ferguson was unable to undertake administrative duties because of dysentery, yet they did nothing to rectify the situation.[11] Moreover, they both left the site of the impending battle for an unknown destination and did not reappear until a week later, when they still did nothing to deal with the 6000 casualties, one quarter of the force involved. Guthrie wrote to Dr Ferguson saying that 'the inhumanity of not leaving a sufficient number of medical officers to deal with the severely wounded rests exclusively on Dr Franck and Dr Taggart'. Guthrie's frank personal letter of criticism of his immediate superior officers was typical of his character (he even demanded their court-martial), for at that time he was only a young regimental surgeon and yet he risked his own military career out of loyalty to his friend Ferguson, whom he thought was likely to be held responsible, and

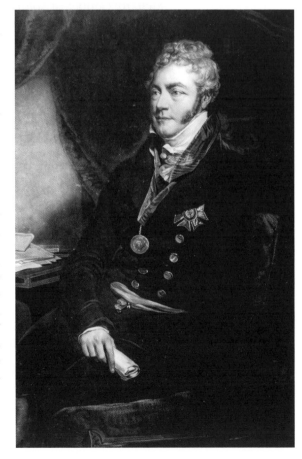

Figure 2.3 *Director–General Sir James McGrigor (1771–1858) (reproduced with permission from the Wellcome Library, London)*

also because of his strong humanitarian concern for the welfare of his troops.

Worse was to follow when Wellesley decided to evacuate the town, withdraw to Portugal across the river Tagus and leave the wounded behind. Franck decided to leave no medical personnel to care for the wounded but to rely on the French (the enemy) to deal with the situation. In the event most of the injured decided to walk back with the retreating army. Many gave up after several days' marching and were assembled in the Convent of Deleytosa, near Truxillo **[6]**, which Guthrie later described as 'the slaughterhouse of the wounded of the British army', because of the lack of medical care and the large number of unnecessary amputations (especially of the arm) which had been carried out.[11] These outspoken comments made Guthrie unpopular with many of his fellow surgeons but his growing surgical and administrative reputation made him worthy of attention. The lack of proper care for those unfortunate soldiers who were hospitalized because of illness or injury was vividly described by Richard Cooper, a soldier who had developed dysentery and had been taken into the convent:

> My case was pitiable, my appetite and hearing gone, feet and legs like ice, three blisters on my back and feet unhealed and undressed, my shirt sticking in the wound caused by blisters ... and worst of all nobody seemed to care a straw for me.

At one time he was in a room without ventilation with 20 other patients, 18 of whom died. He had no soap or towel and survived on biscuits, salt pork and wine.[8]

All army surgeons have extraordinary tales to tell – one such event occurred during the battle of Talavera as Guthrie was about to change the position of his aid post to avoid ricocheting cannonballs. He saw a man running towards him waving his hand and shouting for him to stop. The soldier asked him to examine his head on which a cannonball had bounced. The man pulled off his cap and Guthrie was surprised to see a severe depressed fracture with portions of brain and broken bone mingled with the hair. History does not relate the man's fate.[8] A similar episode occurred just before the battle of Salamanca when an Irish soldier of the 27th Regiment saw a cannonball bouncing towards him and shouted 'Stop it boys' and put his foot in its path. His foot was so severely damaged that Guthrie had to amputate it.[8]

Three more lucky escapes from death

Guthrie became exhausted by the labour of medical and administrative work and developed malaria as the army retreated into Portugal during the autumn of 1809. He was taken by bullock cart from Portalegre to Abrantes and left there to die. At that time it was usual to give bark for these fevers and the Inspector–General, thinking that this would be the last time that he would see Guthrie, stressed the necessity for him to take it; he obeyed, although against his own practice and his feelings. This treatment made him so much worse that he requested the regimental nurse, whom he had fortunately kept with him, to buy half a dozen lemons and to 'slice them into a pitcher of water fresh from the spring. It held two gallons. This he drank during the night with the effect of causing profuse perspiration for several hours after which his fever left him but with feet so swollen and legs so weak as to be unable to walk for several weeks'.[4]

Guthrie returned to England in the spring of 1810 for six months' convalescence prior to returning to Spain later that year with the rank of staff surgeon. During the siege of Badajoz in 1812 he again had a lucky escape from death whilst riding alone outside the town when a cannon was fired at him. He saw the flash and was then astonished when a large round shot passed between his back and his horse's tail. He raised his cap to compliment the gunner on the accuracy of his aim and rode off 'at a good canter'.[4]

During the siege of Salamanca that same year a similar event occurred when Guthrie decided to accompany a young officer of the Welch Fusiliers who wished to promenade in front of the town, wearing a new coat with gold epaulettes and mounted on a white charger, in order to impress the Salamanquinas (ladies of Salamanca). To the French enemy a white charger was indicative of high status and not surprisingly they were both fired upon and almost hit by the French artillery, forcing them to make a hasty and undignified retreat. This same handsome officer was less lucky shortly afterwards when 'he fell from a grape-shot, which entered his abdomen on one side, carrying with it on the other several feet of his bowel which was lying on the ground when Guthrie reached him'.[4]

Battle of Albuhera – 16th May 1811[12]

Albuhera [7] (which means a mill or the village of the mills)[7] was the hardest battle of the war and was won by the English. Massed infantry had poured musket fire into each other at close range all day and the scene of battle was vividly described:

Mr Guthrie placed himself on the plain a little to the rear of the two British divisions of infantry, with the cavalry on the right. It was impossible to keep out of the way of either shot or shell. Assistant surgeon Bolman was struck by one on the chest which went through him. Rain came down in torrents; the lightning was more terrific than the flashes of the guns, the thunder louder; and what with the noise of the cannon, the shouts of the combatants, the cries and moans of the wounded, the outcry and exclamations of the flying Spaniards and the darkness of the day, it might have been thought that all the fiends of Pandemonium were taking holiday. At three o'clock the fight was over and Mr Guthrie found three thousand wounded men at his feet, with four wagons only for their removal and not an article for their relief, except such as might be contained in the panniers of the regimental surgeons.[10]

Guthrie was the senior surgeon during this battle and he operated continuously in pouring rain and under continuous heavy gunfire. His assistant surgeon had been killed and there was insufficient transport to evacuate the wounded to the base hospital 35 miles away. Many of the wounded had lain on the battlefield, 'amongst the dead and the dying, with storms of rain pouring over them'. Although the Spanish were no longer enemies they were ungrateful for the liberation of their country from Napoleon and gave no assistance to the British in dealing with the casualties after the battle.[7] The situation was such that roofing material from nearby houses was stripped for firewood and wooden musket stocks were also collected from the field of battle[13] (see also Chapter 21, cases 36–52). Guthrie and his remaining staff had to operate for 18 hours a day for three weeks – 'from five in the morning until eleven at night their labours were incessant under the most painful circumstances. At the end of three weeks they were nearly worn out; they had obtained the grateful thanks of all those who were about to die'.[10] Guthrie was personally congratulated by the Duke of Wellington for his skill and devotion to duty and was awarded the Albuhera Gold Cross medal (Figure 2.4). It was after this battle that he instituted the policy of ligation of *both* ends of an injured artery to prevent back-bleeding from the distal end, and that he was promoted to the rank of staff surgeon.[13]

The situation after such a battle was well described in *The Lancet*:

It is after a great battle that the work of the doctors begin. Tired, like everybody else with the labour of the previous

Figure 2.4 *Guthrie's Albuhera medal with eight bars for the Peninsular campaign and his Portuguese gold 'Cross of Distinction'(courtesy of Dr Llewellyn Lloyd)*

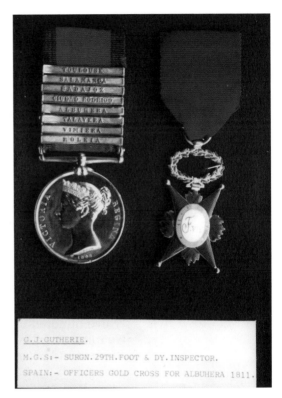

G.J.GUTHERIE.

M.G.S:- SURGN.29TH.FOOT & DY.INSPECTOR.

SPAIN:- OFFICERS GOLD CROSS FOR ALBUHERA 1811.

night and day, the dangers of which they are in great part exposed to unless they absent themselves, they are then called upon to work in a way of which few people have any conception. Nine tenths of the wounded, for the first three or four days, lie on the bare ground; the doctor has to kneel by the side of the wounded man; his back is bent until he cannot straighten himself; his mental and corporeal powers are equally strained to the utmost; and it is not surprising that under such circumstances, wanting almost every-thing, even food, the doctors should often think their own lives worth nothing.[10]

Battle of Ciudad Rodrigo – January and February 1812

The battle of Albuhera was followed by a winter campaign, culminating in the successful siege of the key fortress of Ciudad Rodrigo **[8]** further north, a battle in which Guthrie again had to deal with administrative duties as well as the treatment of the wounded.

Against general army orders Guthrie had decided to retain the injured in the regiments' own mobile hospitals under the care of their own regimental officers rather than send them to general hospitals often 100 miles away. This policy was severely criticized by the Adjutant–General, who noted that Guthrie 'had a greater number of sick with his own division than any other division of the army, contrary to orders which ought to be obeyed'. He also declared that 'if any evil consequences ensued, the responsibility must rest on Mr Guthrie, not on him'.[14] However, McGrigor, who had arrived in Spain earlier that month to replace Dr Franck, himself adopted this new policy three months later at the siege of Badajoz.

Siege of Badajoz – 11th March and 6th April 1812

The successful siege of another key fortress at Badajoz **[9]** followed soon after and Guthrie was in charge of wounded officers and 1200 other men, 'a labour he cheerfully accepted and [he] remained with his division for several weeks as a means of improving his knowledge'.[14] It was after this siege that James McGrigor inaugurated a weekly completion of sick returns by each regimental surgeon (Figure 2.5).

Battle of Salamanca – 22nd July 1812

The battle of Salamanca **[10]**, in which the French lost 14 000 men, including 7000 prisoners, and the English 5200 casualties, of whom 4300 were wounded,[15] left Guthrie 'with many hundred wounded strewed over the field without the capability of removing one', both English and French.[14] After the battle:

'Three hundred unfortunate Frenchman, the worst of the wounded then living, were collected around *[Guthrie]* on the field and when brought into the Convent of San Carlos and laid on the bare ground, the living, the dying and the dead, side by side, the stench was dreadful; never was humanity more outraged. They ate and drank all that Mr Guthrie could give out of their shoes, using the same shoes and caps for all other necessary purposes of life.[14]

The British army was retreating towards the coast and needed the assistance of the Spanish authorities to look after these casualties. But they provided no assistance at all until an impatient Guthrie told them in fluent Spanish and in no uncertain terms that he would leave a letter for the French authorities when they arrived later to collect their wounded comrades. This letter would describe the Spanish authority's inhuman conduct and recommend that 'they hang them to a man'. This had an immediate effect.[14]

RETURN *of* SURGICAL CASES *treated, and* CAPITAL OPERATIONS *performed, in the General Hospital at* TOULOUSE, *from April 10th to June 28th, 1814.*

DISEASES and STATE OF WOUNDS.	Total treated.	Died.	Discharged to duty.	Transferred to Bordeaux.	Proportion of Deaths to the number treated.
Head....................	95	17	25	53	1 in $5\frac{10}{17}$
Chest....................	96	35	14	47	1 in $2\frac{26}{35}$
Abdomen	104	24	21	59	1 in $4\frac{1}{3}$
Superior extremities.	304	3	96	205	1 in 101
Inferior ditto	498	21	150	327	1 in $23\frac{5}{7}$
Compound fractures..	78	29	...	49	1 in $2\frac{20}{29}$
Wounds of spine......	3	3	...	...	1 in 1
Wounds of joints ...	16	4	...	12	1 in 4
Amputations—					
Arm .... 7 ⎫ Leg and thigh 41 ⎬	48	10	...	38	1 in $5\frac{1}{5}$
Total ...	1242	146	306	790	1 in $8\frac{114}{146}$

Wounded Officers 117, not included, making a total 1359, among which thirteen cases of tetanus occurred, and all proved fatal.

Figure 2.5 *Statistical returns of army casualties at Toulouse in 1814 (from Guthrie G.* Gun Shot Wounds of the Extremities, *1815)*

Guthrie's description of a hospital ward after this battle is remarkably frank and compassionate. It also vividly describes what must have been the situation in army hospitals at that time:

> Conceive this poor man, late at night in the midst of others, some more seriously injured than himself, calmly watching his blood – his life – flowing away without hope of relief, one man holding a lighted candle in his hand to look at it and another a pewter wash hand basin to prevent its running over the floor until life should be extinct. The unfortunate wretch next to him with a broken thigh, the ends lying at right angles for want of a proper splint to keep them straight, is praying for amputation or death. The miserable being on the other side has lost his thigh: it has been amputated. The stump is shaking with spasms: it has shifted off the wisp of straw which supported it. He is holding it in both hands in an agony of despair.[16]

It was after this battle that Guthrie introduced the operation of fasciotomy (long incisions through the deep fascia) to relieve the tension of streptococcal infection of the deep tissues of the leg, which at that time was called erysipelas.

In October 1812 Guthrie was posted to Madrid **[12]** and was informed he had been promoted to Deputy Inspector (Figure 2.6), to be responsible for the medical care of seven divisions, a larger force than that under the Duke of Wellington, and also a large military hospital. The army medical board in England refused to confirm this appointment, saying that he was too young and, moreover, they had promoted many men over his head. This angered Wellington, who included this gross injustice in his despatches to England. The effect of this lack of promotion was that when Guthrie left the army two years later his pension was £130 a year (£8500 in 2006) less than it would otherwise have been if this promotion had been confirmed – a situation which continued for 30 years. This rankled Guthrie for the rest of his life.[14]

Guthrie was then transferred to Lisbon and during this lull in the fighting he was able to write articles on 'wounded arteries' and on 'amputations at the shoulder joint', both submitted by his close friend Dr Hooper and published in 1815[14] in Vol. 4 of the *New Medical and Physical Journal*.[1] In the former article he described his policy for the treatment of arterial injuries which he had established at Albuhera, and he emphasized that the Hunterian principle of proximal ligation for an aneurysm was not applicable to these injuries. To illustrate these articles he

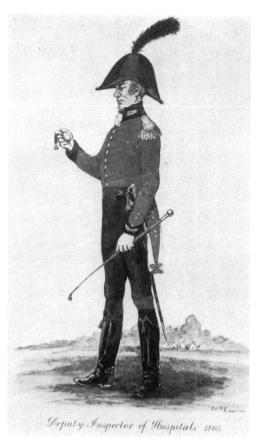

Deputy Inspector of Hospitals 1805.

Figure 2.6 *A deputy inspector of hospitals in full uniform – 1805 (from Cantlie N.* A History of the Army Medical Department *Vol. 1)*

also sent pathological preparations of arterial injuries which he had preserved. At this time the Duke of Wellington was visiting the hospitals in Lisbon and publicly expressed his admiration for Guthrie's work.

In the spring and early summer of 1813 Guthrie was placed in overall charge of the army hospitals in Lisbon and took the opportunity to study the treatment of dehydration, tuberculosis and venereal disease given by the local physicians in civilian hospitals. This led to his opposition on his return to England to the use of mercury for the treatment of syphilis due to its unfortunate side effects. However, he accepted that 'to cure a soldier in a hospital is one thing, and to cure a young gentleman living about town in the usual way young men live, is quite a different matter'.[17]

Santander – 1813

In October Guthrie was made responsible for 800 soldiers who had been wounded after battles at Le Saca and at Vera. Before these battles he had been suddenly surrounded by a group of enemy cavalry under the command of a French officer whom Guthrie had treated a year previously when a prisoner at Salamanca, and who had subsequently been exchanged for an English officer. Guthrie was recognized, immediately released and accepted the grateful thanks of the French officer for the treatment he had previously received.[18] Guthrie remained at Santander [13] for three months until December when he left to join the army in France.

In addition to his medical work Guthrie took over the regimental hospital accounts, which previously had been found to be entirely fictitious. After the submission of accurate accounts for the previous three months the Purveyor–General assured Guthrie that:

> He was known to be the best physician, the best surgeon, the best officer, the best linguist in the army, and that he had now shown himself to be the best accountant, in doing that which no other inspectional officer could have done.[19]

Battle of Toulouse – 10th April 1814

This, the campaign's final battle in France before Waterloo, was the last battle in which Guthrie was involved and indeed it was soon followed by the Peace Conference in Paris. At this battle, thanks to McGrigor's improved organization and Guthrie's untiring efforts, the care of the injured was considered to be adequate – 'nearly all the wounded had every possible assistance and comfort. The hospitals were well supplied with bedsteads, the medicine and materials were in profusion'.[20] Guthrie was also able to say that: 'the surgery of the army was at its highest pitch of perfection it attained during the war, every broken thigh was in a straight splint and the success greater than ever before'.[20,21]

It was only at this last victorious battle that the army had sufficient doctors to manage the expected number of casualties. The hospitals at Toulouse were left 'in the highest order', the English and French (enemy) surgeons visited each other and 'every case of interest was thoroughly investigated'.[22] How typical of the medical profession, then and now.

During the battle of Toulouse the cavalry had been commanded by Sir Hussey Vivian, who had sustained a severe musket ball wound of the arm. Amputation had been advised but this he refused until he could be seen by someone more experienced. Guthrie was consulted and he advised conservative treatment which proved to be successful. Many years later Sir Hussey introduced Guthrie to his second wife on the occasion of his marriage: 'I introduce you to Mr Guthrie, to whom you and I are both indebted for the arm on which you are now leaning'[4] (see also Chapter 8, p. 128).

After this battle Guthrie's earlier observation at Salamanca of metastatic abscess following secondary amputation of infected limbs was confirmed.[23]

Bayonet charges

An interesting observation is made in Guthrie's *Commentaries on the Surgery of the War* concerning bayonet charges, contrary to the general belief in England:

> Opposing regiments, when formed in line and charging with fixed bayonets, never meet and struggle hand-to-hand and foot-to-foot; and this for the very best possible reason, that one side turns around and runs away as soon as the other comes close enough to do mischief; doubtless considering that discretion is the better part of valour.

Small parties of men may have personal conflicts after an affair has been decided, or in the subsequent scuffle if they cannot get out of the way fast enough.[24]

At the battle of Maida (a typical bayonet fight) 'the sufferers, whether killed or wounded, suffered from bullets, not bayonets. It may be that all those who were bayoneted were killed, yet their bodies were never found'.[24]

Medical administration during the Peninsular War

The medical administration during the Peninsular campaign had been very poor and the rectification of this fell upon Guthrie's shoulders until the arrival of James McGrigor as replacement Inspector–General. When the British army had first landed in southern Spain in 1808 the medical stores for the whole army had required only two bullock carts for their transport and none had arrived 'at the place or at the time' that they were required.[22] Guthrie continually complained about this inefficiency of the medical department during the first two-thirds of the war and it was only when the army reached the Pyrenees towards the end of the campaign that its medical department attained an acceptable standard, but sadly only one year later at the battle of Waterloo the administration was again poor.

This lack of organization of the medical services in the British army is described by Cantlie in his account of the Peninsular campaign[7] and confirms Guthrie's continued frustration and irritation recounted in his writings, a situation made so much worse by comparison with the better facilities available to the French wounded which had been organized by Baron Percy (Figure 2.7); in particular, his design for the sprung *ambulances volantes* (see Figure 11.2, p. 173) and stretchers (see Figure 8.3, p. 138). These were staffed by a dedicated medical corps. Likewise, in the French hospitals there had been no reliance on untrained regimental orderlies, a situation which had greatly handicapped the treatment of the British wounded.

Extended personal account of the Peninsular War

In *Compound Fractures of the Extremities* (1838) Guthrie provides a vivid personal account of his experience during the Peninsular War. In fact, despite its title, this historical record occupies most of the book; its surgical content is relatively small, although important. Chapter 3 of this biography comprises abridged excerpts from these extensive personal reminiscences.

An army surgeon's life in the early 19th century

Administrative structure

In the early 19th century the medical services of the army had a Director–General based at the Army Medical Board in Berkeley Street, London, and Inspectors and Deputy Inspectors situated in the theatre of war, under whom were staff (full) surgeons, regimental surgeons and assistant surgeons, in descending order of seniority. Each regiment had a surgeon and a hospital mate (equivalent to a house surgeon), and at the base hospital there would be several staff surgeons (equivalent to a consultant).

Ranks in the army medical service[25] were:

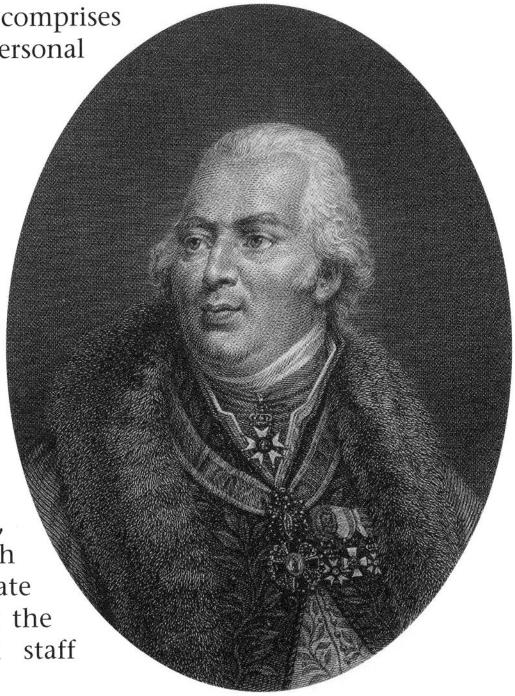

Figure 2.7 *Baron Pierre François Percy, a senior surgeon in the French army and second-in-command to Surgeon-in-Chief Baron Larrey (reproduced with permission from the Wellcome Library, London)*

Title	Status
Hospital mate	Subaltern
Regimental assistant surgeon	Subaltern
Regimental surgeon	Captain
Staff surgeon	Major
Deputy Inspector–General	Lieut. Colonel
Inspector–General	Brigadier

Work in the field of battle

When going into action the regiment was accompanied by a surgeon and an assistant surgeon (Figure 2.8). In the early stages of the war they stationed themselves seven paces (about 7 metres) behind the regimental colours which were always displayed during a battle to identify the site of the regimental aid post. Often they would be identified by a black feather on a cocked hat and they carried a limited supply of dressings for first aid and the control of haemorrhage.[7] After several surgeons had been killed or severely wounded it was realized that this position was too exposed and dangerous, and later in the campaign they were stationed further to the rear. Even so, the regimental surgeon frequently worked in an exposed position close to the actual fighting, and this was graphically described in the second lecture of *Commentaries on the Surgery of the War*, when Guthrie wrote:

> I stationed myself behind a small watch-tower and the wounded were first brought to this spot for assistance. A howitzer had also been placed upon it, being rising ground, and at the moment I was extracting a ball situated immediately over the carotid artery the gun was fired, to the inexpressible alarm of surgeon, patient and orderly, who bolted in all directions. From my hand being unsupported no mischief ensued and the operation was completed as soon as all had recovered their usual serenity.[26]

Likewise, Guthrie said that 'a military surgeon should never be taught to expect any convenience; his field pannier for a seat for the patient and a dry piece of ground to spread his dressings and instruments upon, are all that are required'.[27]

The injuries sustained in these battles were from a sword, from low velocity lead shot from a pistol or musket, or from a 6, 8, 9 or 12 lb shot fired from a cannon.[28] The former frequently remained in the body of the injured soldier whilst the latter could carry away a whole arm, as shown in one of Charles Bell's paintings of a casualty at Waterloo (Figure 2.9). Guthrie always operated on a severely wounded soldier if he thought there was a chance of life being saved. He thought that in this situation an army surgeon had no alternative:

> A soldier ought never to die without surgical aid where there is a chance of its being successful. This kind of case will very much decrease the surgeon's average of success, but he will have done his duty.[8]

The injured often showed remarkable self-control, as demonstrated by Fitzroy–Somerset, an aide to the Duke of Wellington and who was later in command in the Crimean War. As his amputated arm was being taken away he called out: 'Here, bring that arm back! There is a ring my wife gave me on the finger'.[8]

The hospital scene

There are very few descriptions of a hospital after a battle, though such a scene was described by an infantry sergeant after the battle of Waterloo. He wrote:

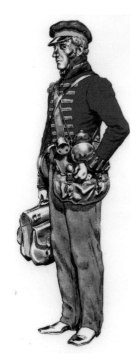

Figure 2.8 *A regimental assistant surgeon in campaign dress during the Napoleonic Wars (reproduced with permission from Worcestershire Regiment Museum, Worcester)*

Figure 2.9 *Left arm carried off by a 12 lb howitzer shell. The axillary artery appears to have been ligated on the battlefield and is clearly visible. The soldier is holding on to a rope with his remaining arm to help himself move into a more comfortable position. The soldier recovered from his injuries (from Crumplin M., Starling P. A Surgical Artist at War. Roy Coll Surg Ed 2005 p. 80. Reproduced with permission from Army Medical Services Museum)*

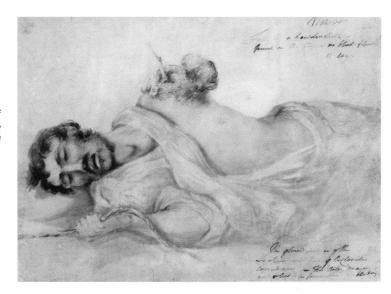

I looked through the grating and saw about two hundred soldiers waiting to have their limbs amputated while others were arriving every moment. It is difficult to convey an idea of the sight or appearance of these men. Their limbs were swollen to enormous size and the smell from the gunshot wounds was dreadful. Some were sitting upright against a wall under the shade of a number of chestnut trees and many were wounded in the head as well as in the limbs. The ghastly countenance of these poor fellows presented a dismal sight. Their eyes were sunk and fixed and there they sat, silent and statue-like, waiting for their turn to be carried to the amputating tables.

A little further on were the surgeons. They were stripped to their shirts and bloody. A number of doors placed on barrels served as temporary tables. To the right and left were arms and legs flung here and there without distinction, and the ground was dyed with blood. The operation was the most shocking sight I have ever witnessed. It lasted an hour *[this is much longer than was usual at that time]* but the man's life was saved. The first cut seemed to be the most painful, after which the operation was borne with comparative indifference or even boredom. When the arteries were taken out all the men said it felt like the application of a red-hot iron.[28]

Presentation to Guthrie from Officers of the 29th Foot Regiment

The officers who served in this corps between the years 1801 and 1809 have presented to Mr Guthrie, their late surgeon, a piece of plate, value 150 guineas *[£9840 in 2006]*, as a mark of their regard and esteem for his personal character, and the high estimation they entertain of his professional abilities displayed by him during that period in the regiment.[6,29]

This very valuable presentation was made 20 years after the end of the Peninsular campaign and demonstrates the regiment's high opinion of their surgeon.[30]

Guthrie's army career in Portugal and Spain – a summary[31,32]

Guthrie had arrived in Portugal in 1808 with the 29th Foot Regiment as an unknown regimental surgeon; he was promoted to be a staff surgeon two years later in 1810 and, again, in 1812 to Deputy Inspector. During the army's advance across Spain he was placed in charge of a new general hospital in Madrid, the administration of which was exemplary, including the supervision of weekly returns from the surgical staff which had been requested by McGrigor, of whom Guthrie was a great supporter and, with justification, an admirer. He was decorated by the Duke of Wellington at the battle of Albuhera for his skill and devotion to duty, and between 1808 and 1814 he personally treated 20 000 wounds. Undoubtedly during this time he advanced the science and practice of military surgery more than anyone since the time of Richard Wiseman (the 'Father of English surgery') in the 17th century.[29] As he said in the Preface to the *Commentaries*: 'The precepts laid down are the result of the experiences gained in the Peninsula, which altered, nay overturned, nearly all those which existed previously'. And in 1855 (again in the *Commentaries*) he said that they 'have been fully borne out and confirmed by the practice of the surgeons of the army now in the Crimea in almost every particular'. Guthrie's rapid promotion had been due partly to his obvious surgical skill and partly to his excellent administrative ability when in charge of the 3000 wounded after Albuhera.

When Guthrie returned to England he was treated as a hero and later he became known as 'the English Larrey'. Baron Dominique Larrey had been the senior surgeon to Napoleon's army, which he had accompanied on most of its expeditions, and he had become revered throughout Europe for his bravery and devotion to duty. Until Larrey's time, the casualties had usually been abandoned on the battlefield and had been attended by camp followers and occasionally by a surgeon. Larrey ignored rank and treated the injured, including any captured enemy, in order of severity.

Another army surgeon, Haddy James, wrote later that he had found the medical work 'grim in the extreme', alleviated only by the heroism of the suffering soldiers.

When one considers the hasty surgery, the awful sights the men are witness to, knowing that their turn on that blood-soaked operating table is next, seeing the agony of an amputation, however swiftly performed, the longer torture of a probing, then one realizes fully of what our soldiers are made.[33]

The Royal Society obituarist well summarized Guthrie's career during the Peninsular War: 'In these fields of action he justly earned the highest reputation amongst the British military surgeons of his time; and all his writings prove that they were to him fields *not only of action but of study*' (author's italics).

Notes and references

1. Cited by Pettigrew TJ. *Biographical Memoirs of Physicians and Surgeons*. London: Whittaker, 1840, p. 1, 10.

2. Biographical sketch. *Lancet* 1850; **1**: 726–36.

3. Guthrie GJ. Introductory lecture. In: *Commentaries on the Surgery of the War*, 5th edn. London: Renshaw, 1853, pp. 7–8.

4. Op. cit. ref. 2, p. 730.

5. Guthrie G. Preface. In: *A Treatise on Gun Shot Wounds of the Extremities*. Burgess and Hill, 1815, pp. v–vi.

6. Everard H. *History of Thos. Farrington's Regiment, the 29th (Worcestershire) Foot 1694–1891*. Worcester: Littlebury, 1891, p. 274, 308.

7. Cantlie N. *A History of the Army Medical Department*. London: Churchill Livingstone, 1974: Vol. 1. pp. 299–301. Also cited by Cantlie from Ross Lewin *With the 32nd in the Peninsula*. London: Simpkin Marshall, 1904, p. 109.

8. Laffin J. *Surgeons in the Field*. London: Dent, 1970, pp. 73–5, 77.

9. Op. cit. ref. 5, 1820, p. 4.

10. Op. cit. ref. 2, p. 731.

11. Op. cit. ref. 2, p. 729.

12. *Albuhera* is often spelt *Albuera* without an *h*. In the first clinical lecture in *Compound Fractures of the Extremities,* p. 2, Guthrie said that if it were not spelt with an *h* 'you might as well spell *London* without a *d*'.

13. Op. cit. ref. 7, pp. 330–1. See also ref. 3, Lecture 12, p. 223.

14. Op. cit. ref. 2, p. 732.

15. Op. cit. ref. 7, p. 347.

16. Op. cit. ref. 3, Lecture 12, p. 214.

17. Op. cit. ref. 1, p. 19.

18. Op. cit. ref. 7, p. 348.

19. Op. cit. ref. 2, p. 733.

20. Op. cit. ref. 3, 6th edn (Philadelphia), p. 146.

21. Op. cit. ref. 7, p. 371.

22. Guthrie GJ. Preface. In: *Wounds and Injuries of the Chest.* London: Renshaw, 1847, p.1.

23. Cule JH. Some observations of Guthrie on gunshot wounds of the thigh during the Crimean War. *J R Soc Med* 1991; **84**: 675–7.

24. Op. cit. ref. 3. Lecture 2, pp. 36–7.

25. Ackroyd M, Brockliss L, Moss M, Retford K, Stevenson J. *Advancing with the Army.* Oxford: Oxford University Press, 2006, p. 32.

26. Op. cit. ref. 3, Lecture 2, p. 33.

27. Bowlby AA. British military surgery in the time of John Hunter and in the Great War. Hunterian Oration 1919. London: Adlard, 1919, p. 25, quoting Guthrie and cited by Moore W. *The Knife Man.* London: Bantam Press, 2005, p. 135.

28. Crumplin MKH. *Trans Hunterian Soc* 2000–1; **59**: 35–6.

29. Biography of GJ Guthrie. *Br J Surg* 1915–16; **3**: 5–7.

30. Watts JC. George James Guthrie, Peninsular Surgeon. *Proc R Soc Med* 1961; **54**: 767.

31. Op. cit. ref. 30, 764–8. A good, short account of Guthrie's service in the Peninsular War.

32. Laffin J. Guthrie, McGrigor and the Peninsular War. In: *Combat Surgeons.* Stroud: Sutton Publishing, 1999, Chapter 8.

33. Op. cit. ref. 8, p. 86. *Surgeon James' Journal 1815* (found by his granddaughter in the loft of his house). Vansittart J. London: Cassell, 1964.

CHAPTER 3

Personal reminiscences of the Peninsular War

*C*ompound Fractures of the Extremities, published in 1838 and summarized in Chapter 19, is in reality a personal record of Guthrie's experience in the Peninsular War. The surgical content, though important, is very minimal. The narrative provides an account of the conduct of war in the early 19th century; of the general lack of organization and the privations of soldiers of all ranks, including officers, whilst on the march; of how the troops were led from the front by senior officers; and of the poor conditions of service during the whole campaign, in particular those of the doctors. It also provides a revealing insight into the life of an army surgeon and the dangers to which he was exposed during the Peninsular War. These personal reminiscences make fascinating reading, despite the loquacity of the author, so frequent in 19th century writing.

There are stories of incredible bravery (narratives nos 1 and 2), two strange illnesses (no. 3), a lucky escape from death and an amusing account of a monk's seduction (no. 4), the plundering of dead soldiers (no. 6), the control of haemorrhage by pressure (no. 10), the logistics of army transport and preparation for a battle (nos 7–9, 11–13), two amusing incidents during the campaign (nos 14 and 16) and the quality, career structure and status of medical staff (nos 15, 18 and 19).

The following are *considerably* abridged extracts from Guthrie's personal account of the Peninsular War.

The bravery of Lieutenant–Colonel George Lake in August 1808

The action of Roliça was an eventful day for many; for none more than for George Lake *[Figure 3.1]*, the Lieutenant–Colonel commanding the 29th regiment. He fell at the moment of victory and, as far as I know, no one

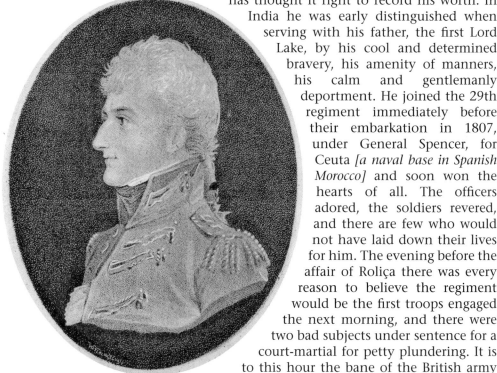

Figure 3.1 *Lieutenant–Colonel George Lake (from Everard H* History of the 29th Foot Regiment *(courtesy of Worcester Regiment Museum)*

has thought it right to record his worth. In India he was early distinguished when serving with his father, the first Lord Lake, by his cool and determined bravery, his amenity of manners, his calm and gentlemanly deportment. He joined the 29th regiment immediately before their embarkation in 1807, under General Spencer, for Ceuta *[a naval base in Spanish Morocco]* and soon won the hearts of all. The officers adored, the soldiers revered, and there are few who would not have laid down their lives for him. The evening before the affair of Roliça there was every reason to believe the regiment would be the first troops engaged the next morning, and there were two bad subjects under sentence for a court-martial for petty plundering. It is to this hour the bane of the British army that there is great difficulty in getting rid of men upon whom neither precept, prayers nor punishment have any effect. There were at that time several in the regiment who had received from four to eight thousand lashes; they were incorrigible on some points but most gallant soldiers. The British army must occasionally be flogged as no discipline could be maintained without it. *[See also the story of Ned in Chapter 1, p. 6].*

Colonel Lake, when he formed his regiment in the evening for the punishment of the two culprits, knew full well that every man was satisfied they deserved it, but he did not say that. He spoke to the hearts of his soldiers; he told them he flogged them not only because they deserved it, but that he might deprive them of the honour of going into action with their comrades in the morning, and that he might not prevent their guard from participating in it. The regiment was in much too high a state of discipline to admit of a word being said, but they were repeated all the evening, from mouth to mouth; and the poor fellows who were flogged declared to me that they would willingly, on their knees if they dared, have begged as the greatest favour he could bestow, to run the risk of being shot first, with the certainty of being flogged afterwards if they escaped.

Early the next day we came up with the French, drawn up in line, the heights of Roliça behind, and covering the main road. They were the two battalions of the French 70th regiment, and the 29th and the 22nd advanced in line to meet them. A line of two deep, either for attack or defence, is peculiar to the British; all other nations attack in column, but British disciplined troops can do what none others can do. We advanced in perfect order with shouldered arms, until the red tufts, nay the very faces of the French line, could be distinguished, Lake and his horse seemed to be prancing with delight.

I was told my place on such occasion was seven paces in the rear of the colours and he seemed to be so much in front. At this moment he turned round, calling out: 'Gentlemen, display the colours' *[the colours of the regiment were always displayed immediately before a fight to encourage the troops for the glory of their regiment, to raise their morale and to help them lose their sense of fear]*. The colours flew, he and the horse had another prance, when he turned again and addressed the line: 'Soldiers, I shall remain in front of you and remember that the bayonet is the only weapon for a British soldier'. The Light Company was ordered to the front, when some of the old grenadiers called out: 'we can do it as well as them, Colonel'. His smile was beautiful in replying: 'Never mind, my lads, let the Light Bobs lather them first, we will shave them afterwards'. A narrow steep ravine seemed the only accessible part and up this Lake, without a moment's hesitation, led his grenadiers on horseback *[Figure 3.2]*. The whole regiment followed, with unexampled devotion and heroism, and gained the summit; but not without the loss of 300 men in the desperate conflict which took place, almost hand-to-hand in the olive grove half way up the hill.

Broken and overpowered by numbers, Lake fell and his soldiers would have been driven down if the 9th regiment had not rushed up with equal ardour, led by no less a gallant soldier Colonel Stewart. The two regiments formed on the crown of the hill. Colonel Lake on horseback on the top of the hill seemed to have a charmed life. One French officer said afterwards that he had fired seven shots at him. Once he seemed to stagger as if hit but it was only at the seventh shot that he fell. It is probable that he was right for he was wounded in the back of the neck slightly; but the ball which killed him passed quite through from side

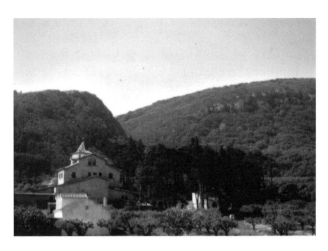

Figure 3.2 *The ravine up which Colonel Lake led his regiment (courtesy of M. Crumplin FRCS)*

to side beneath the arms. The sergeant–major, seeing his colonel fall, stood over him like another Ajax, until he himself fell wounded in thirteen places by shot and bayonet. I gave him some water in his dying moments and his last words were: 'I should have died happy if our colonel had been spared'; words that were reiterated by almost every wounded man.

Colonel Stewart, of the 9th, fell also. He was struck by a musket ball in the belly. I saw him a short time afterwards lying under a myrtle bush and he beckoned me to come to him. 'Our friend Brown', said he, meaning the surgeon of the 9th, 'gives me no hope, pray look at me'. I did so and he saw I had none either. He thanked me and begged he might not detain me from others to whom I could give relief. He died, poor fellow, a few hours after, with the resignation of a Christian and the firmness of a soldier.[1]

An addendum to this account in Major Everard's *History of the 19th (Worcestershire) Foot 1694–1891* (Worcester: Littlebury 1891) records further information concerning this day:

The 29th regiment was at this moment coming up with Lieut. Colonel the Honourable G. Lake at their head, the band playing a country dance, Lake was mounted on a complete charger, nearly seventeen hands high, with a famous long tail, and was dressed in an entire new suit, even his leathers, boots, hat, feather, epaulettes, sash etc. being all new, and his hair powdered and queued, his cocked hat placed on his head square to the front, and, in fact, accoutered in the strictest accordance with the King's regulations.

[After the Colonel had been wounded Major Campbell] immediately went up and expressed a hope that he was not seriously wounded. Colonel Lake lifted his eyes, took Major Campbell's hand which he pressed with all his remaining strength and soon expired. The body was then covered with a cloak and after the action removed for internment. As Major Campbell was passing, many of the wounded called out to him: 'Never mind us, sir, for God's

sake take care of the Colonel'. *[The site of his burial is marked by a stone monument surmounted by a cross (Figures 3.3 and 3.4) and there is also a plaque in Westminster Abbey (Figure 3.5).]*

Sir E. Pakenham – another remarkable and brave man

I know no man of those who are no more, who can be compared with Lake, except Sir E. Pakenham, who was never so animated as before the enemy; the sound of a shot seemed to give him the greatest delight; he snorted it like a racer on the course, and like Lake, he was always the first in danger and the last out of it. Careless of themselves,

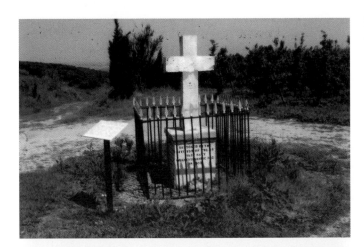

Figure 3.3 *Colonel Lake's grave at Roliça (courtesy of M. Crumplin FRCS)*

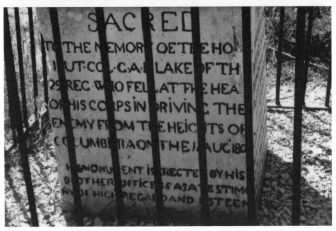

Figure 3.4 *Inscription on Colonel Lake's grave. 'Sacred to the memory of Lieut. Colonel Lake of the 29th Reg., who fell at the head of his Corps in driving the Enemy from the Heights of Columbeira, on the 17th August 1808. This monument is erected by his Brother Officers as a Testimony of their high Regard and Esteem (courtesy of M. Crumplin FRCS)*

Figure 3.5 *Memorial tablet surmounted by a sculpture in the wall of the north–west tower of Westminster Abbey, on the right as you face the exit. 'Sacred to the memory of the Hon. George Augustus Frederick Lake, late Lieut. Colonel in His Majesty's 29th Regiment of Foot, who fell at the head of his Grenadiers in driving the enemy from the Heights of Roliça in Portugal on the 17th August 1808. This stone is erected in his memory by the Officers, Non-Commissioned Officers, Drummers and Privates as a testimony of their high regard and esteem'. It is somewhat difficult to see because of its situation high on the wall and the poor lighting (author's photograph, reproduced with permission from Westminster Abbey, London)*

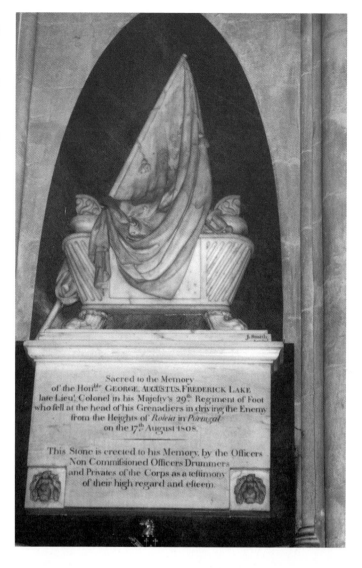

considerate for others, wounded on several occasions, they seemed to forget that such a thing could again occur.

At a later period in the fierce conflicts in front of Vittoria, he lost a friend, an officer of his old regiment the Fusiliers, who was killed by a ball which lodged in his backbone. His widow arrived some time afterwards with four children from Lisbon, alike wanting in friends and of means. Sir E. Pakenham sent me a hundred pounds for her use, desiring me to say it came from a fund in the regiment, to which she was entitled on account of her children. Spare, he said, at all hazards her feelings; they will be greatly hurt if it is offered as a present from me. She does not know to this hour that this money came from Sir E. Pakenham.

I parted from Sir E. Pakenham on the day he started for his last command. On shaking hands I said: 'We now part for the last time; I shall never see you again'. He asked: 'Why say so; what makes you a prophet of evil?' I replied: 'I know you so well that I feel confident you will not be able to hear the first shots fired without being in the affray; you will be killed, I fear, foolishly'. He knew the feeling that dictated this and, in pressing my hand more warmly, he said: 'That I shall fall is possible'. In the front of a regiment which appeared to be failing in its duty, on horseback, with his hat off, he received his first wound. Feeling that he could not sit his horse, he endeavoured to dismount. In the act of lifting his right leg over the saddle, a second shot struck him above the groin, and it was afterwards found had divided the great iliac artery. He fell dead and he kept his word.[2]

Haemoptysis due to a leech and anaemia due to an ingested salamander

A soldier had suffered from bleeding for several days in considerable quantity from the mouth, and neither medicine nor treatment seemed to have any effect upon him. He became greatly emaciated and his death seemed to be inevitably at hand, although I could not find any particular disease about him. On visiting the hospital early in the morning I enquired if he was dead and was astonished at being told he had been quite well for two hours and intended to live, for he had coughed up a leech which there could be no doubt was the cause of the bleeding, inasmuch as it had ceased from that moment. The man rapidly recovered. I was quite aware that in warm countries, in which leeches prevail, they are readily taken up by men and horses in drinking out of puddles, as thirsty animals, whether bipeds or quadrupeds, will constantly do. They are usually what are called horse-leeches, or of that kind which hold on and suck at one end and discharge the blood at the other; but they commonly stick about the lips, mouth and throat, both in men and horses, from whence they are readily removed by fingers or forceps. When they get above or behind the palate they are still usually discovered with a little trouble; and when they could not, I never before or afterwards found much difficulty in dislodging them with strong salt and water injected through the nose, which by its own virtue and that of vomiting had the desired effect.[3]

Dr Robb gave me the particulars of a case which nearly killed a man who had been drinking out of a puddle, or out of a canteen filled from one. The man declared he felt something move in his stomach the instant he had drunk, and from that moment his torments were unceasing, both from pain and from the alarm he felt at distinctly perceiving something trotting up and down his stomach. The man became pale, wan and miserable and would have died in spite of all the means employed for his relief if he had not at the end of about three weeks, vomited up a living animal, the cause of all his misery. The case is so well attested by the medical officers who saw the animal before it died that it cannot be disputed. They say it had four feet and a long tail and called it a salamander, I presume from no medicine having had any effect upon it rather than its deserving that name. It was so large that it nearly choked the man in coming up, so that he was quite satisfied it had grown considerably after he had swallowed it.[3]

Lucky escape from death near Oporto, capture of a gun and the monk who made love to a lady

We marched all night to surprise the French at Albergaria Nova. The wounded at this place passed under my observation but gave nothing of importance. The French had collected all the boats on their, the northern, side of the river, and apparently considered them so secure as not to think it necessary to place a sufficient guard over them. The consequence was that soon after the British troops reached the southern bank of the Douro in Villa Nova, the suburb opposite Oporto, one boat was loosened and brought over. The soldiers immediately embarked, crossed and brought back others, amidst the shouts and vivas of the natives. Sir J. Sherbrooke soon followed with the whole 29th regiment; and the Portuguese boatmen, having procured more boats, ferried me over with my horse. The alarm was perfect. The French, who appeared not to have suspected such an accident, fled, leaving horses, mules and baggage in all directions; every one took to his horse or his heels, and no one thought he could get to Oporto fast enough.

The inhabitants seemed afraid to touch anything themselves but called out to us to seize every horse and baggage-mule we saw as French. Being the only officer on horseback I could ride about and take my choice of lots of loaded horses and mules but I was much too proud to take possession of three or four mules with their baggage. It was not yet considered officer-like to deal in baggage and so I occupied my time in looking for some riding horses, until I lost the British and was overtaken by Sir J. Milley Doyle at the head of the 16th Portuguese, looking for the English. I offered to show him the way as they were only a little before us and placed myself by his side at the head of his regiment.

On turning a corner I showed him the 29th Grenadiers drawn up in line on the rising ground at the end of the road. They as soon perceived us and, after a minute or two, I saw Sir J. Sherbrooke himself face the Grenadier company towards us and to my astonishment they very quietly made ready as if on parade. Sir John and the Portuguese called out it was all over with them, and I thought so myself for, knowing the old grenadiers very well, I took it for granted we were as good as dead. We were too far off to be heard in time, yet close enough to be shot, and it was quite plain they took us for French. I bethought me I had a red round jacket on under my blue undress coat and, as little time was to be lost, I stood up in my stirrups and opened the blue coat as wide as possible, that none of the red one should be lost. The Grenadiers at this moment came to the present; I thought we were gone; when in an instant I saw them irregularly changing to the recover; they knew me and had called out: 'the doctor and the Portuguese'. I never was so delighted in my life and galloped up towards them forthwith. Sir J. Sherbrooke saluted me with: 'By God, Sir, if you had not shown that red jacket I would have sent you all in a second more to the devil'.[4]

From that day the Portuguese never went into action without a white band round the left arm. Shortly after this I accompanied the light troops to the front and had a little skirmish with the French runaways who were making their escape from the end of every street. Some of them brought out a gun but on seeing us and that the road was occupied, they dismounted and left the gun and the four mules that drew it. This I went to the left and seized, but what to do with a gun and four mules I did not know, more particularly after my failure in horse-stealing; so I settled the matter by taking possession of the best mule, which I carried off and it served me very faithfully through the Talavera campaign.[4]

Sir John Sherbrooke must have been a gastronome by his unbounded admiration of the kitchen at Alcobaça. It was, however, a good one and the live fish did swim about in troughs placed from one end to the other on the middle of the table through which the river water constantly flowed; and the gardens were beautiful in the extreme. The padre guardian and the monks were always hospitable. They were obliged in those days by their charter to give a dinner and lodging to every traveller who passed and asked for it, and about three half-pence on parting in the morning, and they received us with open arms on all occasions. The dinner was most joyous, the monarch and people of the respective nations were drunk with enthusiasm. I think I now see the jolly old fellows answering to our three times three with a thousand vivas; but they were not all old and the young ones liked wine.

On one occasion, when Sir J. Sherbrooke dined with them, one of the younger ones was also successful in making love; for the English ladies who accompanied the soldiers were not fastidious and one of them could not resist the solicitations of the handsome monk. He was caught by the soldiers in a situation unhappily for him pas douteuse *[without a doubt]*. They immediately placed him on one shutter and the lady on another and marched them joyously round the cloisters to the great amusement of the populace assembled at the convent to see the British. The next morning he had disappeared; his trial and punishment were summary; he had been sentenced to a slow death on bread and water, in a small stone cell from which he was never to be withdrawn alive. The entreaties of Sir J. Sherbrooke prevailed not. The superior honestly admitted that he would have forgiven the offence at the pressing entreaty of the English general if it had not been so publicly manifested; but that the character of the order was at stake and it must be as publicly known that the punishment had been exemplary.

Sir John kept up a correspondence with the padre who assured him that he and his order, as well as all Portugal, owed everything to his gallantry. Sir John Sherbrooke, with the characteristic feeling of an English gentleman, took him at his word and wrote him back that he placed such implicit reliance on all that he had said that he could not refrain in reply from asking him for the pardon of the young offending monk as the greatest favour he could do him. Sir John Sherbrooke, when he told me this story, declared that he had felt that day to be one of the happiest of his life when he received a letter from the superior enclosing one from the young man thanking him for his life, and stating the horrible imprisonment he had undergone and the utter destitution of hope in which he lay, when Sir John's interference and his pardon were announced to him.[4]

The advantage of regimental hospitals and severe criticism of Guthrie

The Duke of Wellington had shown a strong preference for general hospitals, amounting almost to a prohibition of regimental hospitals. His Grace mentions the extreme difficulty he had to make officers of all ranks obey orders on any subject, each being pleased to think for himself, so that it was not the doctors alone that incurred his displeasure. The question may be justly divided into two parts; one of necessity, the other of choice. If he is in a situation which he knows he is going to leave, he may not choose to encumber the troops on marching with a number of sick or to leave the country studded with small detachments of them to misbehave or act as they please. The establishment of regimental hospitals is forbidden for more than temporary purposes, or for those whose illnesses are not likely to last more than three or four days; the others he sends to the rear by his return food and forage mules, their conveyance thus costing nothing. The disadvantages of a general hospital are that the sick arrive in bad condition when there is no accommodation for them; and they suffer accordingly. The medical officers generally have no particular interest in them, know little of their duties, the wants or the tricks of the soldier, and cannot take the same care of them.

My accumulation of sick at last, however, got me into a scrape. The adjutant–general sent for me to know why I had so many sick and wounded, and what I meant to do with them. I told him that they were much better with me, provided they were not in danger from the enemy, and he allowed me to keep them on my own responsibility. Sir James McGrigor, whom I had seen but twice before, and hardly therefore knew, told me very formally I was the worst officer he had, that I was totally unworthy of any trust and must be sent to the rear where I could do no more mischief. It happened, luckily for me, that there was no one at hand to put in my place, and I was therefore informed that as there was a senior at the siege of Badajoz which had just commenced, I might go there and try and do my duty better when I arrived in the camp. Those of the medical officers who had worked with me at the two previous sieges of Badajoz and at Albuhera, and who knew I had lately done half the duty of the siege of Ciudad Rodrigo, instead of a quarter because no one else would do it; and had nearly killed them as well as myself by pure hard work during the previous year, fairly laughed at me.[5]

The plundering of dead soldiers

I turned my attention to a French officer who had just been brought in. He was bleeding much from a wound in his face and his white waistcoat and trousers were covered with blood. I spoke to him in French, he immediately pulled out his little book of accounts which every French soldier carries, and returned thanks for falling under my care, and gave me his watch and his money as a matter of course and with the view of begging protection. At the first fight at Roliça the kit of the dead soldier remained on his back untouched, until he was buried, and it is but just to say that the British officers taken under the eye of the French were not plundered. But our troops are apt scholars and few dead or wounded escaped plundering after that day, whether friends or enemies; and the progress we made in arts as well as arms was equally great. The contrast between Roliça and Badajoz will be perceived when I tell you that at daylight, after the storming of the town, I saw thirteen officers lying dead on the great breach, stripped stark naked in the night by their own friends or their allies. In such a way does war destroy our noblest feelings.

Two days elapsed before I could find time to seek for my wounded French officer, I then found him without a sous amongst them; they had been thoroughly well cleaned out, although otherwise well treated, and they admitted they could not have done it better themselves. My poor Frenchman came forward to renew his acquaintance, for although I had apparently robbed him, I had still been kind; and kindness begets kindness. You should have seen him open his eyes when I apologised for not having found him before to return his watch and money. They did not believe I was serious but when they saw me place the watch and the doubloons *[French money]* in his hand they could not restrain their feelings. I was an ange de dieu *[angel of God]*, the most beneficent of human beings. I assured them it was only an act of common kindness that every English gentleman would feel himself bound to do.

The day we started *[on a march to Almeida]* it poured as if all the heavens had opened all their watery stores upon us and no poor devils were ever in a more wretched state than we were on reaching Cernados in Portugal. We had intended to cross the river Tagus but the river had greatly filled in the course of the evening. Next morning we took to the mountains by a bridle track and never stopped until sunset. The bullock carts could make little of this, and half way up they were brought to a standstill. What was to be done? After due deliberation it was thought desirable to burn the carts and the baggage. This consisted of twenty complete sets of bedding and a trunk containing the commanding officer's best suit of clothes, which had no business there. At midnight the conflagration took place. I learnt afterwards from a French officer that they were walking off as fast as they could at the same time when they saw the light of this fire which they took for a beacon to alarm the country people in order that they might cut off some of the stragglers.[6]

Transport to Spain in 1808 and landing in Mondego Bay

In December 1808 the troops embarked in transports maintained at great expense and commanded by men who were oftentimes quite incompetent to the charge committed to their care; and the loss of ships and lives which frequently occurred have been usually set down after formal enquiry to unavoidable accident, when, I have little doubt, they really arose from extreme ignorance or negligence.

My last turn in a transport was from Lisbon to Santander, off which port we arrived in the evening, but too late to go in without a pilot; so we lay to, with a good fine breeze on shore, the tiller lashed a lee, and the mate and one sailor to keep watch. At midnight I looked out of my port-hole and saw the ship was making way fast and approaching the shore, and there was a very odd noise from time to time on the deck, as if the tiller was wagging about at its own pleasure. Thither I repaired forthwith and found this to be the case. The tiller had got loose, the mate and sailor were asleep, and the vessel was fast going into Santona, under the guns of which we should have been in another hour.

The army landed in Mondego Bay with the expectation of seeing the enemy forthwith; but no arrangements were made for sick or wounded with the regiments. I went on shore with three days biscuits in a haversack on my back, which contained besides a pair of shoes, two shirts, two pairs of stockings, washing and shaving apparatus and a pocket handkerchief. I was ordered to purchase a mule or an ass for the instruments and medicines by the commanding officer, who could not give me any money to buy it. I have no doubt there were plenty of stores on board ship, but it is the arrangements, and the utter ignorance of the subject, which is ludicrous. Each surgeon should have had a pair of wicker panniers covered with bull-hide and duly filled. It was very unwise to trust on an enemy's country for the supply of animals. The allowance made to the surgeon should be sufficient for him to keep it up, for it should be an animal more than equal to its work and should invariably march before the last section of each regiment and should never be allowed to go to the rear.

When we marched to surprise the French on the advance to Oporto, an order was given for all the baggage animals to go to the rear. I, however, placed the mule with the physic and the entrenching tools in this situation and walked and rode by the side of them. In the middle of the night the general of the division was furiously angry at the order having been disobeyed and desired to know for what reason I dared to have two mules there. I very submissively replied that, as it was understood we were going to surprise the enemy, it was very probable that they might like to fight rather than be taken, and that we might thereby have some wounded, when the surgical stores were wanting. He then desired to know what business I had with the entrenching tools. Now I dared not say that such a thing might happen as the pickaxes being wanted to knock down a wall or for other military purposes, so I very maliciously replied they might be some killed as well as wounded, and it might be as well to bury them. This only made him the more angry and he ordered the mules to the rear. In about ten minutes the aide-de-camp came back to say the general would allow the mules to return.[7]

Before the battle of Toulouse in 1814

When we crossed the river Garonne to fight the battle of Toulouse, the left flank of Fusiliers crossed the bridge of boats first, then the band playing the British Grenadiers, then my two mules, followed by Sir E. Pakenham and myself. Two French videttes galloped forwards, fired two shots over our heads to announce our crossing, and then retired. Times and men were altered and it was well known that a doctor without his apparatus was not much better than a battery of artillery without ammunition. In more peaceful times the medical staff mules may march with the general's baggage, but when there is something to be done they should never be out of the doctor's sight; he should be made to keep them equal to any service which infantry can be called upon to do or mules or horses to perform.[8]

The battle of Vimiera – 21st August 1808
Before the battle

We found the French cavalry patrolling between Lourinha and Vimiera to the great alarm of both the natives and ourselves. They counted two patrols of an officer and twenty men each, one being before and the other on one side of us, and told us they would cut us to pieces if they caught us. I had some twenty old soldiers with me, all of whom I knew well, and two or three subaltern officers of other corps, which were taking advantage of the convoy and whose duty it was to fight. I tied the heads of my second bullock to the tail of the cart which preceded them, and thus continued our march across the country which was open though hilly, and soon satisfied my old soldiers that, with their backs against the bullock carts, they were not to be thrashed by a patrol of cavalry. The pots and pans arrived safe, ready for the battle of Vimiera on the 21st.

The 20th was a beautiful day and I spent it happily with three officers, my messmates, who are all since dead. Captain Gauntlet fell, mortally wounded, at Talavera. He was struck on the head by a ball which cut his hat and carried away a portion of his skull and brain. It ought not to have done this if his skull had been of anything like an ordinary thickness; it was unfortunately, however, as thin as thick cartridge paper used in packing and he lost his life in consequence; he died in my arms. Captain Humfrey was struck on the hip by a cannon-shot at Albuhera which carried away the limbs of two men behind him, and died on the spot encouraging the advance of the regiment for the honour of old Ireland, of which he was a native. The third died in bed. He rode with me the whole fight at Toulouse, and when all was quiet and I was giving directions about my wounded, the French fired their last shell; it burst just over us. It is quite impossible for a regimental surgeon to be out of fire if he does his duty.[9]

The battle

The morning of the 21st dawned upon us in all its brilliance; distant clouds of dust announced the approaching contest; our breakfast of biscuits, water and a bunch of grapes was soon dispatched and we moved to the high ground on the left of the British position. The fight had begun before we got there and the French advance was, as usual, valiant. I met with a wounded officer, whose ball I pulled out of his thigh for three inches, hanging in his shirt like a shilling at the bottom of a purse. Whilst I was doing this he got a crack from a spent ball on his hind-quarter which made him jump, and we thought it advisable to retire into a water course which allowed our heads to be under cover. Shortly after this Sir H. Burrard came on the field but one sight of him convinced me that he was unfit to command an army in the field; he was too large in the waist. If the Government of this country will allow soldiers to gratify their military propensities and serve before the enemy, they must first take care they mortify their gastronomic ones. Lord Byron says: 'I hate a dumpy woman', although the particular dumpy alluded to by him was, I assure you, worth looking at; and I equally hate a dumpy soldier, not that they cannot stand fire but because they cannot stand fever.

General Nightingale's brigade, to which I belonged, formed in line on the brow of hill. The French made a show of advancing across the valley and their officers gallantly set them an example; but it would not do, it was only a straggle and they soon retired.[9]

Control of haemorrhage by pressure

I had cut off two or three legs with the help of my assistant when, on amputating a thigh high up, the tourniquet-buckle broke and it fell to the ground; the bone had just been sawn through and the limb fell with it; the patient was likely to bleed to death. I seized the bleeding end of the femoral artery with the finger and thumb of one hand and compressed the artery in the groin with the other, whilst my assistant put a ligature on the vessel above my thumb. I found I had perfect command of it with each hand and, when we recovered from our alarm, I could not help saying: 'why, what would Mr John Bell mean by frightening us all so by saying it was impossible by ordinary pressure to prevent the passage of blood through the femoral artery?' Thinking, however, that I had met with an exception to the general rule, and that Mr Bell might still be right and I in the wrong, I went into the village of Vimiera the next morning to try the point on another amputation or two. I worked away all day, few people being gluttonous of work, and established that I was right and that Mr Bell had given the exception rather than the rule.

When we came home in 1814 our contemporaries in London knew little or nothing of our improvements. I settled this matter by inviting as many gentlemen as pleased to come to the York Hospital in Chelsea. I took an arm off at the shoulder joint without any tourniquet compression at all and, in order that they might be more than convinced, I allowed the great axillary artery to throw its jet of blood over two or three of them, that they might see how easily and completely it was in the power of my finger and thumb.

Sir Charles Bell *[John Bell's younger brother]*, in his Institutes, lately published, has endeavoured to support Mr J. Bell's opinion by saying that if he were wrong with regard to the principle artery, he was right in saying that the bleeding could not be stopped because the collateral vessels would bleed. But this is merely begging the question; none of these vessels give any trouble.[10]

The retreat from Madrid

My situation *[on the retreat from Madrid]* was more desperate than at Salamanca; the loss of a hospital of several hundred men would have materially injured the reputation of the army. What was to be done? I tried my old expedient of speaking Spanish, only in a more daring way. I armed all the orderlies and convalescents in the hospital, marched them into the principal market-place, and seized a dozen fine large four-mule wagons in the name of the Spanish government. The drivers pulled out their knives at once and swore they would not go. The mob collected around us. I showed them several doubloons and assured them the drivers would be paid; that the British army was about to fight for the safety of Madrid, that the hospital must be cleared to make way for the wounded; and I appealed to the honour of the Spanish nation. It was not in vain; the mob at last cheered me; I viva'd in return and carried off the drivers with their wagons, amidst the acclamation of the surrounding populace.

A British army can march through an enemy's country without doing the slightest mischief but it cannot retreat in a similar manner. Every man that falls out becomes a marauder and commits all sorts of mischief. *[To prevent this]* there are three important personages, the commanding officer, the doctor and the drummer, armed with his cat-o'-nine-tails. If they do their duty a retreat may in general be conducted in an orderly manner I rode with the last of the infantry and saw that no one was left behind.

General Napier has three times commented on the officers of the medical department for negligence *[sic]*. If the country cannot give sufficient pay and allowances for good and able men, it is not the fault of the doctors. If they will not reward them when they do their duty well, who is to blame? If they are refused the same indulgencies, the same rewards, the same promotion as the rest of the army, how can the public expect them to be highly efficient? There is no one else to blame but those who have the absurdity to run human life against a paltry economy of money. The Duke of Wellington's opinion was that the doctors had done their duty well.

I trust you will see the advantages of attending early to other studies, besides physic and surgery.[11]

Advance to the River Douro for the Salamanca campaign

The army advanced to the river Douro, when the campaign effectively commenced. We saw the French army marching down the river and our order was received to move in the morning. We usually breakfasted at half past three so as to be secure of one meal in the day. The infantry, after some skirmishing, crossed the Castillo in their rear and formed in line on the higher ground above; and when the mist of the morning broke and cleared away, the light and fourth divisions found the whole French army was upon them; their troops which had apparently marched away in the evening, having countermarched in the night. This brilliant infantry stood as unmoved as if it faced only equal numbers and checked the French advance. As the morning advanced the British army closed up but not in time to prevent twelve *[French]* guns to bear on the roads by which they must retire. Sir Lowry Cole placed six guns to engage them so as to allow the two divisions to pass under their fire without injury. Distressed by the heat the troops ranged themselves along the bank of the river to drink, and the

French brought up their guns immediately above and over-looking them. The sun shone as a southern sun alone can shine; three divisions of British infantry washed their husky throats almost directly under twenty two guns ready to fire upon them at the least sign. Each waited a move. The order was at last given and the British rose, formed in line two deep as usual and then retired. The French artillery opened.

I had placed myself about a quarter of a mile in the rear with three sprung wagons on a rising ground. The whole shot of the French artillery passed by and over us en ricochet, as the military term it, which means bounding along like a cricket ball. As soon as the troops had passed I trotted down to pick up the wounded. As to the standing corn it was not desirable to loiter too long in that, as there was now nothing between us and the French. If there were any poor fellows there, unable to move, they died of starvation. The French did not fire upon us *[whilst collecting the wounded]* and I was happy in being able to repay them in the afternoon, when, under an almost vertical sun, the French and British infantry came into contact. The infantry could hardly drag one leg after the other; yet, when nearly worn out, Sir Lowry Cole advanced in line to the charge. The French stood firm and it was for a few minutes doubtful which party would turn tail and run away. They were now so close as to be almost able to cross bayonets – a thing so often spoken of but so seldom done – when the French turned and walked off across the river.

Our people were quite unable to follow; they had done their best in walking up to them but they could go no further. Some of the French were unable to move and fell into my hands; and I went forward and called to them across the stream to send for the wounded soldiers. Several officers and men came forward immediately, without arms, and you cannot conceive how we complimented each other. The doctors worked all night and we got them all off for Salamanca before daylight.[12]

The battle of Salamanca

Before the battle

I set off in the evening with all the mules we could unload of their bread, corn and spirits to take them out of Salamanca. It was night and the rain came down in torrents, the lightning flashed as closely as if it would strike one to the earth, my horse would not face it and I did not know where the troops were. An officer's servant passed, saying I had no chance of finding the division, although I might find the French. I thought it wiser to go with him and trust to the kindness of the clergymen and the ladies who sheltered themselves under his protection on these occasions. The two ladies were young and had their husbands with them. We all partook of supper and parted apparently regardless of the morrow.[13]

During the battle

The distant sound of a gun during our early breakfast banished the roses from the cheeks of the ladies and brought my horse to the door. Many of the worst cases of the stragglers of the cavalry and infantry were brought to me and between three and four hundred French, in the same desperate state. I foresaw that I should soon be in a predicament unless I exerted myself. I ordered all the medical officers and all the medical establishments to join me, and the commanding officers obeyed without a murmur. Sir James McGrigor could do little beyond acquitting me of blame, for the Spaniards promised everything, but as usual did nothing. They had given him the St. Domingo convent and this he delivered over to me, with permission to badger the Spanish junta as much as I pleased in his name. I could speak French better than any of them and Spanish quite as fast, and I knew their ways too well to speak English. We complemented each other in good Castilian about Spanish honour and humanity, British valour and sufferings, until they declared there was nothing they would not give me. Every cart in Salamanca should go out forthwith for my wounded, every house should find a bed until my hospital was completed. I made them furnish the convent. In two days mine was the pattern hospital; everybody wondered, but nobody found out that this was all done by speaking French and Spanish – that physic and surgery had nothing to do with it.[13]

After the battle

My poor Frenchmen were now my care. I had obtained an empty convent for them but the junta would give me nothing but promises. These poor fellows, although little given to praying, assured me they prayed for me and that, if there was a God in heaven, of which some few of them seemed to have a doubt, their prayers would be registered in my favour. Some months after the affair of Elboden I rode over the ground and found the skeletons of those who had fallen. I was curious in looking at the death wound in each; and in only one case out of twenty odd did I fail to see the broken bone which had been implicated in it. Some of these must, I fear, have died of starvation. The sun and rain had bleached the bones the vultures had picked clean.[13]

The poor treatment of a young doctor in the army, and the episode of the pigs

The first appointment a young man receives at 22 years of age is that of a hospital assistant, in which situation he is worse treated than any costermonger's donkey in Westminster; for the donkey is fed, cleaned and lodged; but the doctor must find these conveniences of life for himself and that is not always so easy for a man who has no money in his pockets.

The Commissioner–General provides him with as much meat, bread and wine as ought to last him three days on the road. Having no money to buy a mule he sends his trunks to the stores where they are soon very cleverly plundered of everything valuable, and starts with a small sack on his back containing a clean shirt and a new pair of shoes. My friend may be attached to a party of bullock cars or mules going up to the army with stores and if this should happen he will have a chance of saving his baggage and getting something to eat, but bullock carts travel only at two miles an hour, so that having ten or twelve miles to travel he is out for twelve or fourteen hours under a burning sun or heavy rain. If he escapes after ten or twenty days of this work, it is only to set off again on a similar travel or to take charge of a large number of sick and share the dangers of a crowded hospital. The cemetery called English at Ciudad Rodrigo contains all that remains of twenty or thirty one of these gentlemen, the victims of distress and disease.[14]

I remember one of these young men who had just come up from Lisbon; the village was full of troops, and as the rank of a hospital mate is the lowest of commissioned officers, his lodgings were none of the best; his bed on the ground floor, an equal distance between the peasant and his wife, and an old sow and a dozen pigs. The peasant, who rose at the dawn of day, woke him. The doctor was indignant at being thus disturbed out of a sound sleep and signalled that he would not get up. The peasant was more vociferous and urgent with tongue and signs that he should shift his position; he looked, as the doctor afterwards said, like a talking sign-post. The matter, however, was soon adjusted, a horn was heard to sound, the peasant tore his hair in despair, out jumped the lady pig right on the back of the sleeper and then sprung out of the door, followed by all her family, to join the swine-herd who was thus collecting them according to ancient custom at the end of the village for their day's pasture in the adjoining field and on the banks of the river. In the evening, at sunset, he thought he would stand at the door and catch the soft but cool breeze that is always felt at that hour. He was thinking of home, for it was just the hour at which he used to steal from the shop where he was apprenticed and take a quiet walk down to the bank of the Thames to enjoy the evening breeze and study the muscles on the naked men who appeared like so many demons emptying coals out of the coal-barges. At this moment he heard the sound of the swine-herd's horn. On looking down he saw the old lady pig, followed by all her family, coming right at him, full tilt, accompanied by all its neighbouring pigs who lived beyond him. In an instant she was between his legs. Only conceive my doctor, with an old sow six feet long by two feet wide, in such a position, his fate was as inevitable as your's would be in a similar situation – over he went, bumped his nose against her tail and rolled covered with blood under the rest of the family who bolted over him into the stye.[14]

The poor quality of some junior surgeons

Circumstances and accidents such as I have related rendered it very difficult to procure good qualified surgeons for the army *[who]* could not be found qualified to kill or cure by commission, they thought it right to take those of an inferior description and give them only a warrant, as they do to boatswains and gunners on board ship. One poor fellow having called to report his arrival, I desired him to sign a paper descriptive of his qualifications. This I found he could scarcely do, the letters very much resembling pot-hooks. I therefore sent him to live at one of the fever hospitals, to do duty for a few days until I might see what he was made of. Two days after going to this hospital at six in the morning I found him in a little alarm. A soldier had been brought to him, he being the officer on duty for the night, riotously drunk; and in order to keep him quiet, he had him tied to the four corners of the first bedstead he could meet with, and having thus got the man on his back recollected he was warranted to do something in physic, he therefore gave him a good dose of tartar emetic, believing his stomach ought to be emptied; but never thinking or not knowing, that a man could not advantageously vomit on his back. He was found suffocated two or three hours afterwards.[15]

Guthrie's own unfortunate experience as a more senior doctor

Perhaps, gentlemen, you may think those doctors who were higher in rank fared better *[Figure 3.6]*. I will give you an example of my own history. I bought a horse and a mule, hired a servant and set off to follow the army to Coimbra. On the fourth day at Rio Mayer, the fellow finding I kept too sharp a watch to permit him to rob me of all I had, ran away with one of my two blankets and my dinner. I was now in a happy state with a horse and mule to clean and nothing to eat. The country was desolate, dead horses, asses and men lay about in all directions and there was little to be obtained of any kind. My assistant surgeon presented me with a blanket he said he could spare. It was almost as fatal a gift as the shirt of Nessus. From that time I ceased to sleep, my flesh seemed to be creeping and crawling all night, I became spotted all over, and wondered what could be the matter with me. On arriving at Coimbra I was sent to the house of a padre, the clergyman of the parish. *[His niece kept house for him]*. She was rather good looking and about five and thirty years of age, which in Portugal constitutes a rather elderly lady. I spoke Portuguese tolerably well and was very

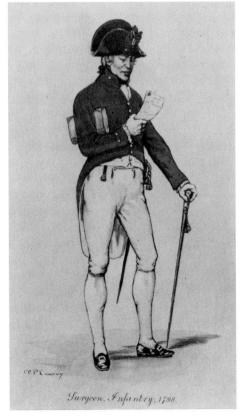

Figure 3.6 *A surgeon of infantry in 1798 (from Cantlie N. A History of the Army Medical Department Vol. 1. Reproduced with permission from the Wellcome Library, London)*

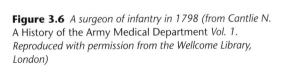

civil to boot and they were both pleased to delight in me. I could tell them the news and could understand their complaints about the French; and they gave me in return an excellent dinner and a very good bed in which I slept soundly for the first time for three or four days. On mentioning this in the morning to my kind hostess, she assured me by a very significant motion of the thumbs, that she knew the cause of the evil and begged to have my little stock of bedding delivered over to her. On coming home from a morning perambulation of the town she met me in an ecstasy of delight, assured me she had my blankets hanging in the sun all day, and that those fleas which had not hopped out her servant had duly destroyed. She further assured me that they were as long each as her nail.[16]

At the battle of Albuhera

In due time I crossed the country and joined the fourth division of infantry near Olivença. I arrived just after sunset, without knowing more than one individual of the whole. It rained in torrents with little hope of its termination; there was nothing to do but to dismount, place one's back against a tree to which the horses were tied and await patiently dinnerless the approach of another day; and no one who had seen my condition in the morning would have pointed me out as the man who, in a short few days, was in the field of battle at Albuhera, to be the arbiter of the lives and limbs of hundreds of his fellow-creatures.

In the middle of the contest I dismounted and had just placed the bridle in the hands of an orderly when a cannon-shot passed between his head and mine. I could not help asking him if his head was on, nor of laughing outright, when, with the most soldier-like gravity he wheeled to the front facing me, touched his cap, and hoped also my head was safe. At the battle of Salamanca the fourth division found itself under the heaviest fire of the enemy. The troops were ordered to lie down under the fire of twelve heavy guns, to which we had only six light ones to reply, and I halted a little in the rear to make my arrangements. As it was plain we were in for a good pelting the general sent his aide-de-camp, Captain Roverea, to ascertain where I had fixed the field hospital, that the wounded might be directed upon it. I was at this moment going to the front and saw my friend Roverea approaching, when my horse stopped and ducked, a sort of gambol that I did not think he was warranted to make from the quantity of corn he had eaten. This motion was explained in a moment; a twelve-pound shot, which he had seen but I had not, ploughed into the loose ploughed field a few feet before him, covered us both with dirt, and hopped calmly but irresistibly over my shoulder. Roverea was so white in the face that I thought he must be wounded; he said he was not, and eagerly enquired if I had seen that shot pass. I said I had and nearly felt it too. He had been shot in the head at Albuhera; his skull had been fractured and, when delirious, he had thrown himself out of bed and thought he owed his life to my kindness. He fell honourably, and for his rank, gloriously, shot through the same side of the head in front of Pampeluna.

After the battle I found myself without conveyance, without stores except those that the panniers of the regimental surgeons contained, and encumbered with near 3000 wounded in the village of Valverde. The doctors all worked as no men ever worked before, the toil was incessant, we thought ourselves happy in the improvement of many around us, and that our reward would follow in the approbation of the higher authorities. *[The higher authorities, however, had been told maliciously and untruthfully by an unknown informer that the wounded had been neglected. The Adjutant–General later realized that these accusations were false]. [Guthrie concluded]* 'Mais revenons á nos moutons' *[an idiomatic expression often used in France, which signifies, when duly translated into English, 'stick to your proper business'].*[17]

The lack of status of an army doctor

I have pointed out to you the miserable and desolate state in which the medical officers, not attached to regiments, are situated in a campaign. These poor creatures suffer in a manner it is quite deplorable to think of, and which is a disgrace to the character of the country. If an unhappy wretch of a doctor has to travel two-thirds of the day, generally on foot, at the tail of a cart of any kind, shivering and wet to the skin, without food, without scarcely a dry change of clothing, with no one to help him in the common necessaries of life, how can he attend to his sick and wounded? It is impossible. Self-preservation is the first law of nature. He must ascertain where he is to eat and sleep, how his clothes are to be dried, to seek food for himself and his beast, if he has one, and to do everything to live himself, except attend to his professional duties. On his arrival at the halting place he ought to see his people housed, put to bed if possible, and give directions for their food, make up their medicines, see them administered, bleed them if necessary, or dress their wounds. A man under a burning sun may do this for two or three hours more if he has a hope of a tolerably comfortable place to rest himself in, or of something to eat, but not otherwise. At night he should again visit his sick and arrange for a move shortly after daylight next morning, when all these duties are to be repeated before the march is begun. No man could do it and the sick have been neglected whenever the doctor was unequal to the duties.

There are two ways of proceeding in order to enable the junior medical officers of the army to do their duty to the sick and wounded committed to their charge. One is by giving them an allowance for a servant, and by giving them a soldier–servant in addition, on service. The second mode of proceeding is by much the best, viz., of appointing three assistant surgeons to each regiment on active service. A young man taken into the army at 21 years of age, which I hope will soon be the age at which he can obtain his diploma as a surgeon, knows nothing of the management of the sick or of providing for them in any way; nor of the character and tricks of the soldier, however good his classical and general attainments may be, in addition to his professional knowledge. He is comparatively inefficient. The assistant surgeon of a regiment learns the duty of a soldier in addition to that of a doctor, and a military surgeon ought to know one just as well as the other.[18]

The varying experience of army surgeons and their career structure

I remember a village in which three regiments were quartered in the sickly season in the autumn when fever prevails. Three rows of hillocks marked the last resting place of the dead on earth and my attention was attracted to one row much shorter than the other two. I found, on enquiry, that the regiments were very much of the same strength and quite under the same circumstances. The doctors were equally able; two were men entering rather on the middle period of life, the third was a very young man and perhaps the worst doctor of the three; but the short row of tumuli belonged to him. I was very desirous of making this out, and after visiting all the hospitals and quarters I ascertained the reason. He was the best soldier, if not the better doctor.

His hospitals were in better order, the material was more perfect, the labour bestowed on every part, except in physic, was greater, and five per cent of human life was the saving and the result. I never saw it otherwise.

A staff surgeon who has not been a regimental officer has this kind of duty to learn; and if he tries it a little late in life, he rarely learns it, and from five to ten per cent loss of human life is the consequence. It was the custom at the commencement of the last war to appoint gentlemen who had influence at home to the offices of staff physician and surgeon, totally overlooking the merits of those who were serving and had therefore just claims for those appointments. This error has been corrected but the situation of the staff officer has not been improved as it ought to have been. He is gazetted a staff surgeon but as the medical officer can hold no direct military rank or command, a relative rank is given him, which is of use only as it regulates his quarters, his baggage, his pension for his widow, his prize money, his horses etc. When promoted, it is natural to think he would then gain something as all other soldiers do; but no, he is to have no servant but is allowed five shillings a week to find one. In the meantime he is appointed to a duty which in the field he can hardly do well, without four animals and two servants, a proportion allowed to every staff-officer of the military branch.

The staff surgeon should always be promoted on account of his knowledge of anatomy, medicine and surgery. He should therefore be promoted for his merit, and should feel that he has gained something as his reward. So far from this being the case he will find his expenses increased, his means being rather diminished, his comforts greatly reduced. The office of staff-surgeon is, therefore, one that nobody wishes to have. And then those gentlemen are generally too old or too idle for any severe or active duty. The last assistant surgeon promoted to a surgeoncy with whom I am acquainted was 26 years an assistant, and it is not very uncharitable to suppose, that at 50 odd years of age he may be unequal to the duties he may have to perform. I have no hesitation in saying that any such person will be unequal to the duties of a regimental surgeon before the enemy. I shall not enlarge on this subject, but merely remark to you that the medical and surgical duties of the Peninsular war were done, when they were well done, by men from 20 to 35 years of age. An elderly man must be an indifferent operating surgeon unless he is in the constant practice of his profession.

Of the senior branches of the medical department I shall only say that they are worse treated than the juniors, but my old and able friend Sir James McGrigor understands this subject better than I do, and will, I hope, be able to improve their situation. There is no man who has more love for his profession, more kindness of heart, a greater desire to act fairly and honourably to every one, but he is without the power of granting promotion except to very few.[19]

References

1. Guthrie GJ. *Compound Fractures of the Extremities*, 1838, pp. 2–4.
2. Ibid. pp. 5–6.
3. Ibid. pp. 46–7.
4. Ibid. pp. 47–8.
5. Ibid. pp. 49–51.
6. Ibid. pp. 30–2.
7. Ibid. pp. 24–6.
8. Ibid. p. 26.
9. Ibid. pp. 26–8.
10. Ibid. pp. 28–9.
11. Ibid. pp. 63–4.
12. Ibid. pp. 59–60.
13. Ibid. pp. 60–3.
14. Ibid. pp. 9–11.
15. Ibid. pp. 11–12.
16. Ibid. p. 12.
17. Ibid. pp. 12–14.
18. Ibid. p. 19.
19. Ibid. pp. 20–2.

CHAPTER 4

Battle of Waterloo and patronage in the early 19th century

G uthrie returned to England in 1814 and tried to establish himself in London. He said in his often dramatic style that he had been 'placed on half pay [a pension], with a month's notice to quit, somewhat like a turned-off footman, and was obliged to seek for other employment'.[1] He had 'placed his all' on this ambition and 'had to await the result'. He joined refresher courses at the Great Windmill Street School of Anatomy organized by Charles Bell and Benjamin Brodie (Figure 4.1), and also at the Westminster Hospital, the Lock Hospital (a charitable hospital for venereal disease, 1746–1952), the Charterhouse Infirmary for Diseases of the Eye and the lectures by Abernethy at St Bartholomew's Hospital. These lectures inspired him to become an author and a teacher. However, his recent army experience in the Peninsular War had made him realize that all these eminent surgeons were out of date and this stimulated him to write his first book entitled *A Treatise on Gun Shot Wounds of the Extremities* in 1815. 'He thus brought himself up to the level of knowledge of the day; and it is a part of his character deserving of our approbation that he has never failed to do so on all points connected with his profession.'[2]

Recall to the army

In 1815 Guthrie was recalled to the army as hostilities had begun again in Europe. At the end of the Peninsular War Guthrie had expressed his 'regret that we had not had another battle in the south of France to decide two or three points in surgery which were doubtful. I was called an enthusiast and laughed at accordingly. The battle of Waterloo afforded the desired opportunity'.[3]

Figure 4.1 *Certificate of attendance at the Great Windmill Street School of Anatomy, designed and signed by Charles Bell in 1825 (reproduced with permission from Royal College of Surgeons, Edinburgh)*

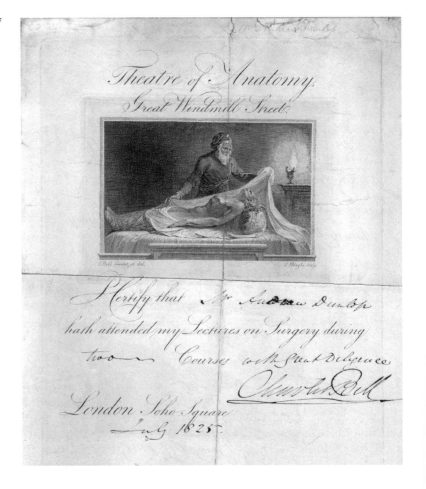

On the outbreak of hostilities Guthrie had declined an offer made by Lord Hill, Sir Thomas Picton and Sir Lowry Cole to join their staff and live with the other officers without any expense to himself in army quarters.[2] But his old friend James McGrigor, who had just been appointed Director–General of the army, wished him to serve again for six months. This he declined as it 'would have been destructive to his prospects in London' and he did not wish to lose more time in establishing himself in civilian practice. He therefore offered himself for three months, but this also was unacceptable to McGrigor, who thought that 'it was too short for the interests of the public'.[2] Guthrie said that he 'had hazarded nearly all he had on his success in London, he could not accept the offer made to him of employment, or the solicitations of many kind friends, high in rank, to accompany them, although he promised to rejoin them in case of accident'.[4] After the battle of Waterloo, however, Guthrie decided to go for four or five weeks 'like other amateurs, without rank, pay or any appointment'[1] 'to establish his opinions on certain points in the management of war wounds which required further confirmation'.[2] This was with the encouragement of McGrigor, who said he could consider himself on full pay and on active service, but without administrative duties.

Guthrie, Bell, Hennen, Thomson and others embarked at Dover on 28th June 10 days after the battle, and arrived in Brussels two days later.[5] Guthrie stayed in Brussels and Antwerp for three weeks as a consultant adviser and visited only the severest cases;[1] he himself only operated on two patients in Brussels and none in Antwerp.[1] 'The whole of the department at Brussels and at Antwerp received him [Guthrie] with every possible kindness, placed themselves and their wounded at his disposal and did everything he desired'.[2] They carried out his every suggestion. Guthrie wrote that the officers in both places had received him in a manner to which he could not do justice.

> There was not a mother, wife or sister of a badly wounded officer at Brussels whose knees were not bent to me, not a father or brother whose hat was not off and to the ground. I was as poor as a rat in those days, but my opinion was not to be purchased; no one presumed to think of such a thing; now that I am not so poor a man *[written in 1830]*, and my opinion may be more valuable, every one thinks he does me a favour who gives me one or two guineas for it. Perhaps it may be so. I was then, however, more gratified in working for nothing than I am now for money. All the senior officers of hospitals offered to send to London any of their bad cases that I could obtain permission to bring over.[1]

The battle – 18th June 1815

The battle of Waterloo had commenced at 11.30 am and was over by 8 pm, by which time there were 40 000 casualties (dead, dying and wounded) spread over two square miles (Figure 4.2). There was only minimal transport to deal with the situation and many casualties had to endure hunger and thirst as they lay on the battlefield for several days in a hot June.

> Some kept themselves alive by eating the flesh of the dead horses which lay around in thousands, their carcasses polluting the atmosphere until Prussian soldiers compelled the local villagers at bayonet point to dig huge pits and bury not only the horses but the decomposing bodies of

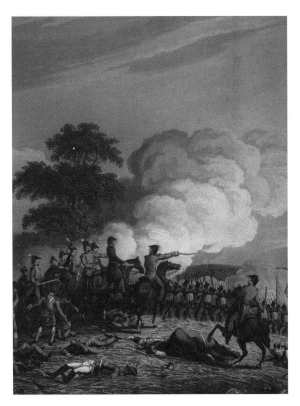

Figure 4.2 *Battle of Waterloo – the commencement of the grand charge made on the French at about 7 o'clock (from Crumplin M., Starling P. A Surgical Artist at War 2005)*

the dead. A visitor to Quatre Bras noted in his journal: 'coming from Waterloo passed forty wagons of wounded crying out'. The men had been in cottages and not able to be removed before. Many died instantaneously; others were in a putrid state – a kind of living death. Every wounded man who could somehow make the long journey of twelve miles to Brussels did so on his own feet, on horseback, or in any kind of vehicle, but for most of the lying cases it was not until the following morning that any aid was possible. Sprung wagons, carriages and carts of all kinds were used to convey the cases to Brussels but it took four days to clear the wounded from Mont St. Jean. A field hospital had by then been set up in the village but until it opened the wounded just continued to die *[Figure 4.3]*.

Every house in Brussels sheltered the injured men and a week after the battle they were still uncounted. Additional orderlies were supplied … but there was no lack of voluntary assistance for delicate women waited upon them and dressed their hurts – every door was open to receive the wounded. Patients were showered with gifts of food and wine. Five large hospitals in the capital were quickly filled and many more wounded were sent off by canal barges to civil hospitals and hotels in Antwerp. Unfortunately the spare hospital beds at Bruges, Ghent and Ostend could not be made use of because of lack of transport'.[6]

In addition to these Waterloo casualties there had been 2380 wounded from the Quatre Bras skirmish three days previously.

Medical services after the battle

After this battle the army medical services were again in disarray; they were grossly understaffed and poorly trained. Most of the Peninsular War doctors had returned to civilian life and very few of those remaining had had any real battle experience. Guthrie wrote,

Figure 4.3 *Battle of Waterloo. The wounded are removed from the battlefield in wagons and the dead are stripped and buried (from Howard M Wellington's Doctors 2002. Reproduced with permission from the Wellcome Library, London)*

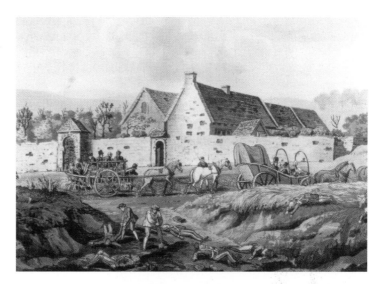

'The confusion during the first few days need not be described' and he was horrified to find that the assistant surgeons, some of whom had served at Toulouse, 'were doing everything that they should not have done'. Moreover, as Guthrie was not on the army payroll and therefore not in charge, he was unable to counteract their incorrect treatment. They did, however, express 'the regret they felt that he should see them doing what they themselves knew he would not approve'. In extenuation they said that they were 'overwhelmed with work, were half dead and could not do more. Their apologies were offered without any word from me, and merely from their own sense of right and wrong. Flemish surgeons had been hired and amateur surgeons had flocked over from London and nothing could recall the irretrievable mischief insufficient care had occasioned in the first few days'.[7] This was the situation when Guthrie and Charles Bell arrived from England to take charge.

Charles Bell (Figure 4.4) reported that 'all the decencies of surgical operations were soon neglected; while I amputated one man's thigh there lay at one time thirteen all beseeching me to be taken. It was strange to feel my clothes stiff with blood and my arm powerless with the exertion of using my knife'.[8] He carried out 146 primary amputations with 40 deaths (27% mortality) and 225 secondary amputations with 106 deaths (47% mortality). Guthrie noted that the greatest problem was compound fractures of the femur and he estimated that two-thirds of these patients died and only one-sixth survived with a useful limb; if the fracture was above the middle of the femur they would all die from septicaemia or shock.

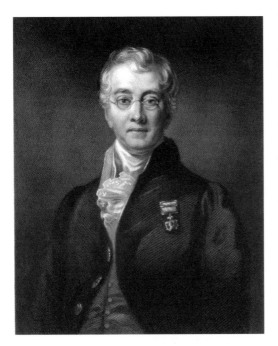

Figure 4.4 *Sir Charles Bell (1774–1842), surgeon to the Middlesex Hospital. Known for his paintings of battle casualties after Waterloo (reproduced with permission from the Wellcome Library, London)*

John Hennen, a staff surgeon who assisted Guthrie in the hip amputation described below, and who wrote *Important Points in the Practice of Military Surgery* in 1818 following his extensive experience in the Peninsular War, had himself treated many of the Waterloo casualties, one of whom was Sergeant Tuittmeyer of the German Legion whose arm had been taken off by a cannon shot (Figure 4.5). Following this injury the sergeant had ridden upright 12 miles into Brussels and reported to St Elizabeth Hospital – an incredible feat of stoicism for a wounded man. A short length of humerus had remained and this was removed just distal to the head of the humerus.[5] Hennen later became Deputy Inspector of Hospitals but died of yellow fever in Gibraltar in 1828, where he is remembered by a memorial stone.

Three operations

After the battle of Waterloo Guthrie carried out three successful operations, two in Brussels and one in London, and these confirmed his leadership in British surgery and his courage as a surgeon.

Amputation at the hip joint

He performed the first successful amputation at the hip joint on a French prisoner, François de Gay – his earlier attempts and also those of Larrey and Dupuytren had been unsuccessful; moreover, Dupuytren (the eminent French surgeon) had declared the operation to be impracticable and that more distal amputation was the only possible treatment. De Gay had lain on his back for four days unable to move and had survived by drinking water from a puddle.[9] A gunshot wound over the greater trochanter had entered from behind, had shattered the head of the femur, which had become separated from the shaft, and had exited anteriorly about four inches below the groin. Charles Bell had also seen the patient and had advised:

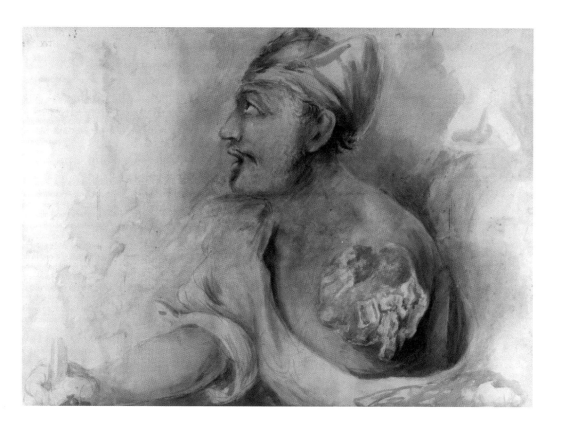

Extraction of the head of the bone only, and do no more. Mr Guthrie's proposal is to amputate the thigh at the hip joint. If the bone be taken out there is a great cavity and suppuration certainly; but by this means the shock and violence will be saved. I fear the shock of so great an injury, especially as now the wound cannot be cut off, and its injury must be superadded to that of the incision. The man will readily allow of my proposal but not of G's. However, next day he said that he would consent. In the meantime I was forced home by business. I had some officers to see.[8]

Figure 4.5 *Sergeant Anthony Tuittmeyer, whose arm was taken off by a cannon shot. The axillary artery is visible and was ligated on the battlefield. Painting by Sir Charles Bell (from Crumplin M., Starling P. A Surgical Artist at War 2005)*

At operation 19 days after injury no tourniquet was used, as digital compression of the femoral artery against the pubic bone was Guthrie's preferred technique (the operation is described and illustrated in *Gun Shot Wounds of the Extremities* 1820 – see Chapter 10, p. 165). The soldier was later able to walk up to three miles, his 'wooden leg being thrown forwards by an exertion of the muscles of the trunk'.[10] Guthrie thought that the success of this operation had depended on the speed with which it was performed, not so much because of restriction of the inevitable haemorrhage but rather because of the lack of shock associated with the procedure.[11]

After this operation Guthrie persuaded the Duke of York to write to Marshall Soult (the French commander) to request the French authorities to provide residence for the soldier in the Hôtel des Invalides in Paris (a residence for battle casualties similar to the Chelsea Hospital in England) – this was accepted.[2]

It is interesting and ironic that this successful operation should have been done on a French prisoner, an operation which Baron Larrey himself had attempted several times without success.

Was this operation really the first successful amputation at the hip joint? English publications all give Guthrie the credit for this operation and this is probably correct, though Dible, in his biography of Larrey (Figure 4.6) in which he quotes extensively from Larrey's own *Memoires*, states that this operation was performed on a French soldier in Russia and that the patient survived for three months.[12] Larrey had always been an advocate of this procedure and may or may not himself have carried out a successful operation. Larrey's description of the injured soldier operated on by Guthrie is worth including:

> One of our own soldiers had been brought in with the English wounded, with his right thigh almost completely shattered by a cannon ball and needed amputation at the ilio-femoral joint. I made bold to suggest this to the English doctor who was present during my visit and to commend the patient to my honourable confrère M. Guthrie, whom I was unable to meet as I had to return to Louvain *[for family reasons]* urgently. The operation was performed by this celebrated surgeon a few days later.[12]

Peroneal artery ligation

A German soldier received a musket ball injury with the posterior entry wound below the head of the tibia. Two weeks later severe haemorrhage occurred from the wound and this was controlled by a tourniquet. Amputation had been considered, as the current accepted treatment was to ligate the main artery proximal to the injury – a procedure that often led to distal gangrene and therefore amputation, especially if the limb itself had also been wounded. Guthrie considered that careful observation and examination of the limb would usually indicate which artery had been injured and that a local exploration of the wound might enable proximal and distal ligation to be performed, with

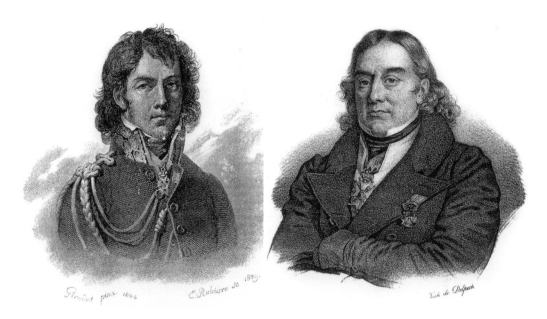

Figure 4.6 *Baron Dominique Larrey (1766–1842). Surgeon to Napoleon's Imperial Guard.* Left, *c. 1804.* Right, *in later middle age (reproduced with permission from the Wellcome Library, London)*

preservation of the limb in many cases This procedure became known later as 'Guthrie's bloody operation'.[2]

Guthrie cut through the calf muscles and ligated the common peroneal artery rather than ligating the more proximal common femoral artery. 'The operation [was] difficult because of slough', he said, 'the artery [was] not identified but blind ligature with a curved needle above and below stopped the haemorrhage'.[13] This operation had been attempted by Dupuytren, who had declared it to be impracticable.[17]

Removal of a musket ball from the bladder

Guthrie used a newly designed instrument introduced through the urethra to remove a musket ball from the bladder – an injury which previously had always been considered fatal due to subsequent infection unless a dangerous open operation was performed. The patient was transferred to York Hospital in London as Guthrie had been due to return to England and he wished to supervise the patient's aftercare. The operation is described in detail in Chapter 8, p. 135.

Return to London

James McGrigor had arranged for these three patients to be transferred to York Hospital, Eaton Square, London, where there was an army medical school[14] and where such cases had never been seen before, either in London or Paris.

The Waterloo visit had cost Guthrie £40 (£2624 in 2006) and he therefore applied to be placed on full pay until he had recouped this loss of earnings. McGrigor replied:

> My good friend, if I do this for you it will be called a job, and no one would be more sorry for it than yourself. I will answer for it you will not fail of success and you will not long want the money. If however, you like to work without pay, and you think it will be an assistance to you as I cannot employ an officer of your rank in London, I will give you two large clinical wards in the York hospital, and you shall have all the worst cases that come from every quarter.[4] *[McGrigor's enthusiasm for controlling army costs was well known.[15]]*

This offer was accepted. It enabled Guthrie to finalize his views on the treatment of war wounds and to provide bedside instruction to illustrate his lectures. He remained in charge of these two wards for two years until their removal to Chatham, and he provided his services gratuitously.

Guthrie commenced a series of lectures on battle wounds which he gave without payment for over 20 years to all officers of the public services. After the first course in 1816–17 he was presented with a silver cup worth 50 guineas (£3280 in 2006), with the following inscription:

> This inadequate but sincere memorial of the admiration of the great professional ability, and sincere respect for his private worth, is presented by the officers of the medical department of the navy, the army and the ordnance, who derived instruction from his lectures, and happiness from his friendship, as they venture to hope for life.[4]

After Guthrie's death the cup passed to his daughter Anne, who passed it over to Henry Power FRCS, who had been a student under her father. In 1919 it was in the possession of Power's son Sir D'Arcy Power (1855–1941), the eminent Bart's surgeon and medical historian.[16,17] Where is it now?

Guthrie's departure for Waterloo had offended his only two private patients, even though his absence was only to be temporary, and they both vowed never to speak to him again.

But his honorary work at York hospital in treating the seriously wounded provided evidence of his surgical skill which rapidly became known and led to an early increase in his earnings from private practice.

Patronage in the early 19th century

The place of patronage in medicine in the 19th century is extensively discussed in a recently published book, *Advancing with the Army:*

> The patron played a key social role in an era in which medical education was undergoing a sea-change. ... Patronage and philanthropy were indissolubly linked in the 18th century.

This continued into the following century.[18] Thus it was that Guthrie gained his medical education under the patronage of Mr Rush.

Patronage continued to play an important part in a surgeon's career and throughout the first half of the 19th century it was important to know the right people. Furthermore, for those without eminent connections or wealth, the army medical service was well recognized as being a stepping stone to a later civilian career and an improved social status, particularly between 1793 and 1815 when 100–200 surgeons a year were being recruited.[19] Thus the army medical service provided a window of opportunity for those who lacked family finance or contacts or even those from a humble background, and this may have been a factor in Guthrie's decision to join the army, for it provided good pay and the chance to meet the right kind of people. England was still a place where this was important.[20] Director–General McGrigor was a clear example of this; he was the son of a tacksman in Strathspey, Scotland, with a name which was still proscribed only a few years earlier, and yet he died a baronet worth £25 000 (just over £1½ million in 2006).[21]

On his return from the Peninsular War Guthrie's lack of wealth made his continuation of patronage important in order to establish himself in London, even though he had made many influential contacts during his army career. He was a man of great potential, a man who was determined to reform the medical profession, which at that time was riddled with nepotism: Guthrie was determined to make good. As Yearsley said in a lecture to the Guthrie Society at the Westminster Hospital in 1892: 'starting in civil practice, he found it, as many have done since, a struggle of no little severity and, in spite of his brilliant success in Spain, he seems to have been but little recognised'.[17] A recent biography of Sir Astley Cooper, an eminent contemporary of Guthrie, emphasizes the importance of patronage and describes how influential it was in his own career.[22]

Guthrie dedicated his first book on gunshot wounds to the Duke of York, Commander-in-Chief of the Armed Forces, in what would now be considered obsequious and effusive language (see Chapter 10, p. 161); and the fifth edition of his *Commentaries* was dedicated to Lord Hardinge, Commander-in-Chief to the British army, concluding with: 'His Lordship's very obedient and faithful servant'. His book on *Operative Surgery of the Eye* was dedicated to the Dukes of Wellington and York, in recognition of their support for the founding of the Westminster Ophthalmic Hospital. In 1840 Guthrie wrote to the Duke of Gordon, with whom he had served in the Peninsula, to thank him for a box of grouse in the following effusive letter, at the same time dropping names:

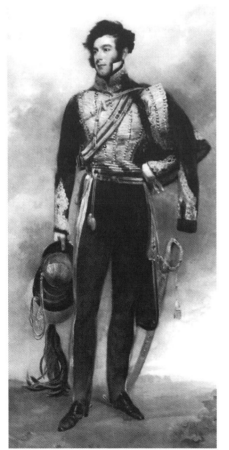

Your Grace was so good as to direct a box of grouse to be sent to me in August but I was unfortunately out of town, having allowed myself this year three weeks with my Lord Panmure at Brechin, which is the reason I did not return my many thanks to your Grace's kindness in thinking of me.[23]

But this was the norm for the time and Guthrie was not alone in this. McGrigor, whom Guthrie admired and whose friendship he valued, also took advantage of patronage, for the late Georgian and early Victorian era was a society in which a knighthood, election to the Royal Society or even a ticket for the Caledonian Ball depended on contacts. Patrons were essentially facilitators and everyone who hoped for promotion or success had to join the patronage game, if possible with dedications in books or pamphlets listing the recipient's full list of titles and honours, followed by tributes to the man.[24]

Figure 4.7 *Lord Chandos, later the 2nd Duke of Buckingham, in the uniform of Commander of the Buckinghamshire Yeomanry (reproduced with permission from the National Trust, Stowe Landscape Gardens)*

This continued throughout the 19th century and Guthrie had little alternative but to follow suit on his return to London.

Loan to Lord Chandos

In 1844 Guthrie lent the improvident Duke of Buckingham £12 000 (£787 620 in 2006) at 4% interest. The Duke assured Guthrie that when his son Lord Chandos (Figure 4.7) came of age later that year the debt would be secured by a mortgage on part of his estate. Though the Duke was very much in debt he promised to assign three life policies to Guthrie as guarantee for the loan. The son was appalled at his father's extravagance and, with other creditors, compelled his father to correct his financial affairs, with the result that the family property was made over to Chandos, on the condition that a schedule of debts was paid. However, the son had inherited his father's talent for embezzlement and the debt did not include the £12 000 loan. Guthrie only discovered this omission when he found that he had not received the loan's half-yearly dividend. Meetings were arranged and Guthrie thought that 'Buckingham and Chandos, father and son, were acting cordially together as their manner implied, for the preservation of the honour of the family of even Royal descent'. He had no inkling of anything like reservation or deception. Matters dragged on but the debt was never repaid.[25-27]

References

1. Guthrie GJ. *Wounds and Injuries of the Arteries,* 1830, p. 60.
2. Biographical sketch. *Lancet* 1850; **1**: 733.
3. Guthrie GJ. Preface. In: *Commentaries on the Surgery of the War,* 5th edn. London: Renshaw, 1853, pp. v–vi.
4. Pettigrew TJ. *Biographical Memoirs of Physicians and Surgeons.* London: Whittaker, 1840, pp. 6–8.
5. Crumplin MH, Starling P. *A Surgical Artist at War.* Edinburgh: Royal College of Surgeons of Edinburgh, 2005, p. 37, 82.
6. Cantlie N. *A History of the Army Medical Department.* London: Churchill Livingstone, 1974, Vol. I, p. 390.
7. Guthrie GJ. Preface. In: *Wounds and Injuries of the Chest.* London: Renshaw, 1848, para 4.
8. Bell C. Cited by Crumplin M, Starling P, ref. 5, p. 3, 41, and also by Guthrie D. *A History of Medicine.* London: Nelson, 1945, p. 268.

9. Crumplin MH. *Men of Steel*. Shrewsbury: Quiller Press, 2007, p. 300.

10. Editorial. Guthrie GJ. *JAMA* 1967; **200**: 408–9.

11. Guthrie GJ. *A Treatise on Gun Shot Wounds of the Extremities*. Burgess and Hill, 1815.

12. Dible JH. *Napoleon's Surgeon*. London: Heineman, 1970, p. 130, 242.

13. Guthrie GJ. Case of wound of peroneal artery successfully treated by ligation. *Med Chir Trans* 1816; **7**: 330–7.

14. *Lancet* 1853; **2**: 290.

15. Ackroyd M, Brockliss L, Moss M, Retford K, Stevenson J. *Advancing with the Army*. Oxford: Oxford University Press, 2006, p. 40.

16. Grimsdale H. George James Guthrie. *Br J Ophthalmol* 1919; **3**: 148.

17. Yearsley PM. George James Guthrie. *Westminster Hosp J* 1892; p. 4. (A lecture to the Guthrie Society on 9th June 1892.)

18. Op. cit. ref. 15, pp. 149–51.

19. Op. cit. ref. 15, p. 16, 150.

20. Op. cit. ref. 15, pp. 27–9.

21. Op. cit. ref. 15, p. 19.

22. Burch D. *Digging up the Dead. Uncovering the Life and Times of an Extraordinary Surgeon*. London: Chatto and Windus, 2006.

23. Op. cit. ref. 15, p. 248.

24. Op. cit. ref. 15, pp. 200–4, 308–9.

25. Op. cit. ref. 15, p. 267.

26. *Stowe Landscape Gardens*. National Trust, 1997, pp. 80–2.

27. RAMC Special Collection 1759/6 Wellcome Library.

CHAPTER 5

Return to civilian life

George Guthrie (Figure 5.1) had served abroad for 14 years. When he returned to England in 1814 he had little money and no prospect of a future inheritance, but he had made numerous friends whilst in the army and was not unduly concerned about his ability to establish himself in London. He bought a small house in Jermyn Street and a year later in 1815 moved to No. 2, Berkeley Street. In 1835 he purchased the two adjacent old houses, Nos 4 and 5, then the offices of the Army Medical Board, and built a large house in which he lived until his death.

He had found it difficult to penetrate the medical establishment in London, for he had few contacts outside military circles and most hospital appointments were made on the basis of nepotism rather than on merit. What should he do, for he was unable to obtain in the near future a post in a voluntary hospital as an entry into private practice? And, moreover, he had been placed on half pay as an army pension,[1] reduced still further because of the lack of recognition of his promotion to Deputy Inspector on the grounds of his youth. An adequate salary was important at this time as he had not yet established himself in London and, furthermore, he wished to start a family with the wife he had married in Nova Scotia. After the battle of Waterloo he was offered a knighthood but he declined this honour as he had been unable to save any money, and if anything should happen to him he considered that 'my lady might be an inconvenient title for a poor woman'.[1]

Westminster Ophthalmic Hospital

In 1816 Guthrie noted that in London there was little systematic instruction in diseases of the eye and insufficient provision for their treatment. So, one year after the battle of Waterloo and with the encouragement of James McGrigor, the aid of Lord Lynedoch and under the auspices of the Dukes of York and

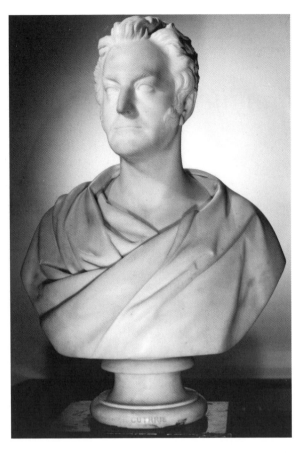

Wellington, he founded the Westminster Ophthalmic Hospital situated in King William Street, Strand, next to the old Charing Cross Hospital. Until suitable premises had been found Guthrie saw patients in his own home. Guthrie and Dr Forbes were appointed surgeon and physician, respectively, to the new institution 11 years later in 1827. For many years the hospital was sustained by Guthrie's early friends from the Peninsular War, and he himself donated £142 (£9188 in 2006) towards its funds during its first 15 years.[2]

Several months later *The Lancet* criticized the hospital's management, following which Guthrie threatened to sue Thomas Wakley, its editor. Forbes wrote to say that if there were court proceedings he would be unable to withhold certain unfavourable evidence and therefore Guthrie withdrew the action. A further dispute between Forbes and Guthrie concerned the treatment of two patients. Abusive letters were exchanged and Forbes challenged Guthrie to a duel, which he declined as he considered it an inappropriate way to settle a dispute; however, his young assistant, Hale Thomson, who was even more hot-headed than Guthrie, had used insulting language to Forbes and accepted the challenge, which was fought with pistols on Clapham Common. Three shots were exchanged on 29th December 1827. Neither party was injured, the seconds intervened and Forbes declared his honour satisfied.[3]

As a reward Guthrie endeavoured to have Thomson appointed to the staff. At first this was not accepted by other members, who questioned his surgical competence, and it was only achieved when he agreed to marry the hospital's treasurer! Thomson was a strange personality and disliked by his colleagues; surprisingly, several years later, he opposed the appointment of Charles, son of Guthrie, his chief supporter, to the Westminster Hospital.[4] Later, he lost much of his money in a speculation in the silvering of glass, became depressed and died from an overdose of chlorodyne in 1860.[5] Forbes subsequently published two pamphlets containing all the correspondence.

Guthrie remained in sole charge of the hospital until some of his duties were taken over by his son Charles as assistant surgeon in 1838.[6] Subsequently the hospital was called the Royal Westminster Ophthalmic Hospital and in 1928 it moved to Broad Street, Bloomsbury,[7] but is now closed following its amalgamation with Moorfields Hospital in 1955.

The foundation of this hospital had caused a great deal of ill will and jealousy amongst a few senior members of the London medical profession, leading to acrimonious and probably libellous articles in *The Lancet*, so vituperous that Guthrie again threatened to sue the editor for defamation. This threat he later withdrew, partly because of possible 'erroneous testimony' and adverse publicity[1] and partly because he had received an apology from *The Lancet*, whose editor had realized that the accusations were completely undeserved.

In 1819 Guthrie published a book on the creation of an artificial pupil, an operation which he had pioneered in England. He reviewed extensively the work of European surgeons, discussed the indications for the procedure and described his own technique in detail (see Chapter 12). Four years later, in 1823, the book was incorporated into a much more comprehensive 517-page book on eye surgery, the demands for which required a further edition four years later (see Chapter 13). Two hundred pages were devoted to cataract surgery. In 1834 he published a third eye surgery book devoted entirely to cataract surgery, for which he was one of the first to stress the advantage of *removal* of the opaque lens rather than the traditional technique of 'couching' (displacement of the lens backwards and to one side with a needle) (see Chapter 17). This was contrary to the current medical opinion at that time. He described in very great detail his operative technique because he felt that previous English publications had not described all the problems which might be encountered and 'did not quite tell all'.

Westminster Hospital

In 1823 Guthrie was elected assistant surgeon to the Westminster Hospital when a new vacancy was created as a mark of 'their estimation of his surgical reputation and character', and this must have satisfied his immediate surgical ambitions. He was elected full surgeon four years later in 1827 and remained on the staff until his resignation in 1843 to make way for his son Charles as assistant surgeon. He was shrewd, quick, active, robust and voluble to a fault and his tongue made enemies.[8]

His appointment brought such a wind of change to the hospital that he practically disrupted the whole edifice, for he had two faults – he was tactless and somewhat of an opportunist.[8]

In 1834 Guthrie and others wished to establish a medical school, a site for this was purchased and the school opened. Guthrie delivered the introductory lecture and did so for the next four years until succeeded by Benjamin Phillips, surgeon to the hospital. Controversy concerning the school continued, however, due to professional jealousy between members of staff and the school closed.[5] In 1853 a new school was established and on the 10th October Guthrie presented to it a signed copy of *Injuries of the Head Affecting the Brain and The Anatomy and Surgery of Inguinal and Femoral Hernia*.[8]

Presidency of the Royal College of Surgeons of England and election to the Royal Society

Over the next 20 years Guthrie was five times Vice-President and three times President of the Royal College of Surgeons of England (known as the Royal College of Surgeons in London until 1843) (in 1833, 1841 and 1854), during which time he insisted on protocol rather than the backward and secretive manipulation of executive procedures that had been followed in the past. He was scrupulously fair in his dealings with his colleagues and also had a deep sense of justice. He radically changed College administration (see Chapter 6).

In 1827 he was elected a Fellow of the Royal Society, being described as 'a gentleman well versed in several branches of knowledge and a zealous promoter of science'.[7] He had been proposed by his friend Sir James McGrigor for 'his constant activity in publishing his knowledge and opinions on all the questions which he had the opportunity of studying'.[9]

Military surgery – Guthrie's main interest throughout his life

Guthrie had revolutionized military surgery during the Peninsular War and had paved the way for its more rational treatment, and this continued to be his main interest throughout his life. He did not respect established opinion unless it agreed with his own experience and he was courageous in trying out new treatments. But this was not without considerable opposition, for the opinions of Hunter and the Bell brothers, John (Figure 5.2) and Charles (see

Figure 5.2 *John Bell (1763–1820) (reproduced with permission from the Wellcome Library, London)*

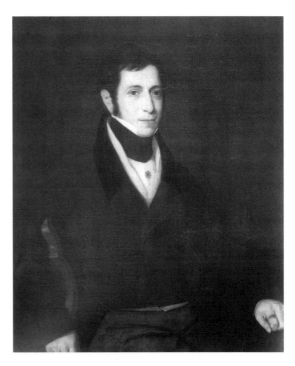

Figure 4.4, p. 66), had been universally accepted, such was their reputation in the early 19th century. But their opinions had been based on only very limited battle experience, far less than that of Guthrie, and were often indefensible. Guthrie later wrote that it had cost him the labour of seven campaigns and 30 years of teaching to refute the opinions of Hunter and Bell, such was their great prestige and influence.[10] The two most important points on which they differed were the question of primary (early) or secondary (after 24 hours or later) amputation for severe limb injuries, and the necessity for distal, as well as proximal, ligation of an injured artery (see Chapter 8). Guthrie was also a pioneer of conservative surgery, as shown by his advocacy of excision of a localized bone fracture rather than amputation and his exploratory operation for an arterial injury (see Chapter 8, pp. 128 and 130).

It is very evident from his writings that he had kept most detailed records of the patients he had treated during the Peninsular campaign.

In 1853 in the introductory lecture to the *Commentaries* Guthrie wrote:

> To use the words of my much lamented friend Sir Astley Cooper, the art of surgery ... received from the practical experience acquired *[in the Peninsular War]* an impulse unknown to it before.

Military administration and teaching

During the Peninsular War Guthrie had constantly complained about the poor administration of the army medical department due to its division into so many different offices and their lack of central coordination. Partly as a result of his efforts, but mainly due to those of McGrigor, the medical board was abolished after the battle of Waterloo. McGrigor had been appointed its first medical director and the situation improved. Sadly, only one year later at the battle of Waterloo, the administration was still poor 'because the system was wrong', and this situation persisted until the time of the Crimean War. In 1848 Guthrie wrote in the Preface to *Wounds and Injuries of the Chest*:

> The same result has followed the four great battles fought in India, the same loss of life, the same succession of human suffering, the same loss to science. The surgeons were overwhelmed by the extent of their labours. It was utterly impossible for them to give due attention to even half the wounded.
> *[Finally, he said:]* The cause is well known – the remedy is in great part attainable. The evil remains; *[and concerning administration he added:]* The same evils will always follow if the same system is pursued.

Colonel Ballance, of the Royal Army Medical Corps (RAMC), wrote in 1917 that he thought that Guthrie may have had more of a scientific bent of mind than his French contemporary Larrey:

> *[Guthrie said]* Surgery is never stationary and surgeons of the present day must continue to show that surgery is as much a science as an art. I believe nothing in surgery until fairly tried and found to answer. A knowledge of the practice of physic is inseparable from the practice of surgery if the patient is to receive that assistance which the art and science of medicine in its most comprehensive sense can grant.[11]

Reform of the army medical services continued to be Guthrie's major interest throughout his life. A young officer, the son of one of Guthrie's friends, had been wounded in the leg by a musket ball, leading to considerable haemorrhage:

> A tourniquet was applied instead of the required operation being performed and he was sent on board a transport at Balaklava. The leg mortified as a matter of course and was amputated. He died, an eternal disgrace to British surgery, or, rather, to the nation which will not pay sufficiently able men – and therefore employs ignorant ones – the best they can get for the money.[11]

In 1840 Guthrie and McGrigor together gave evidence to the Royal Commission on Promotion in the Army and Navy, as they were both frustrated by the lack of promotion prospects for serving army surgeons. They both emphasized that unless the service was properly treated it would fall apart. Guthrie, in particular, exaggerated the situation and declared that the army surgeon was the 'most neglected officer in the service', which required 'medical officers of good administrative knowledge and best professional ability. Such men can only be obtained by adequate remuneration, rewards and honours'.[12]

Guthrie acted as an unpaid teacher to army surgeons, with whom he had considerable correspondence during the whole of his civilian career. His first course of lectures was in October 1816 and these he continued to give *without payment* for almost 30 years. However, he noted that 'it is thought proper to employ a gentleman of high character to teach the veterinary surgeons how to cure the horses of the army; and surely something of the same kind should be done for the men'.[11]

In 1855, one year before his death, he was as zealous as he had been 40 years earlier in 1815 for the sound administration of the army medical department.[13]

Commentaries on the Surgery of the War

Guthrie's monumental book *Commentaries on the Surgery of the War* (see Chapter 11), his *magnum opus,* which also appeared as a series of articles in *The Lancet,* was first published in 1815 immediately after the battle of Waterloo, and ran to six editions, the last in 1855, with an American edition in 1862, especially produced for the American surgeons during their civil war (1861–5). The book comprised over 600 closely printed pages and followed the Hunterian tradition of being based on accurate clinical observation of patients and also extensive use of Guthrie's own anatomical dissections and post-mortem studies. It covered all aspects of limb and blood vessel injuries, head, chest and abdominal wounds, together with amputations, and it included 423 aphorisms concerning the treatment of these injuries. Perusal of these aphorisms shows that, in addition to the treatment of limb and abdominal injuries, he had remarkable insight into the management of penetrating head injuries, the signs and significance of brainstem compression (with an early description of the Babinski reflex), and also the physiological effect of a large haemothorax and of cardiac tamponade.

The *Association Medical and Surgical Journal* (the predecessor of the *British Medical Journal*) was most complimentary of the work and 'heartily commended this attractive and commendable book' to its readers. It stated that 'among military surgeons Guthrie stood second to none'. His obituary notice said that his work on military surgery was 'a monument to the clearness of his head and the vigour and perseverance with which he pursued anything which he undertook'.[14]

Guthrie's influence continued up to the next generation of surgeons. *The Surgeon's Pocket Book* by Major Porter, Assistant Professor of Surgery at Netley,[15] was published in 1875 and was based largely on Guthrie's *Commentaries*, which by then had become the most important surgical textbook in the British and American armies. Surgeons were also advised to read Guthrie's *Pamphlet on the Hospital Brigade* (see Chapter 8, p. 139), which included his instructions to army surgeons.

Guthrie was not averse to criticizing some of his colleagues' opinions – 'the operations were highly honourable to the gentlemen concerned as proving of their anatomical knowledge. The principle on which they acted I presume to condemn'.[16] What was most important was that the patients should receive the best possible treatment.

Literary labours and work as an author

Guthrie (Figure 5.3) had a prodigious capacity for writing, shown by his authorship of 12 books on war injuries and eye surgery, two of them bestsellers, with several of them revised in later editions in the light of more recent knowledge and experience. In the Introductory Lecture in *Wounds and Injuries of the Arteries*, Guthrie complained bitterly about the lack of profit from medical publishing and about the commission he had to pay to the printer and the retailer of his books (see Chapter 15, p. 212), a situation still applicable in 2007. He wrote well and lucidly, although in a loquacious style characteristic of the 19th century. His books always included a large number of detailed case histories, clinical observations and post-mortem findings. Furthermore, they included many happy turns of phrase ('unremitting attention in the use of the stethoscope' in case 69, *Injuries of the Chest,* and 'died as much of his doctor as of his wound' in the Introductory Lecture in the *Commentaries*). His descriptions of urinary retention and bladder rupture are especially graphic and memorable (see Chapter 18, p. 235). His two most important books (*Commentaries on the Surgery of the War* and *Wounds and Injuries of the Arteries*) were made compulsory reading for army officers after the battle of Waterloo, and Empress Alexandra directed that two of his military books be translated into Russian for use by the Russian army and for which Guthrie was presented with two diamond rings.[17]

In his writings it is clear that he had a great admiration for John Hunter (Figure 5.4), even though he disagreed with some of his conclusions, and he usually referred reverently to 'Mr

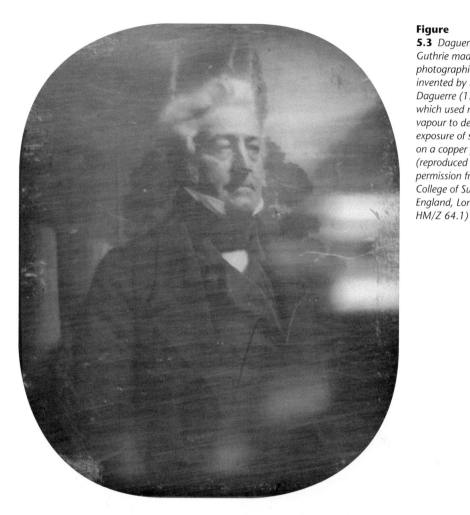

Figure
5.3 *Daguerreotype of Guthrie made by an early photographic process invented by Louis Daguerre (1789–1851), which used mercury vapour to develop an exposure of silver iodide on a copper plate (reproduced with permission from the Royal College of Surgeons of England, London, RCS HM/Z 64.1)*

Hunter', rather than plain Hunter. This admiration is especially obvious from reading *Wounds and Injuries of the Arteries,* in which he emphasizes that the researches of Hunter had anticipated most of the observations made later by his contemporaries and successors[17] (see Chapter 15). It is also apparent in his Hunterian Oration (see Chapter 14). In the Preface to *Gun Shot Wounds of the Extremities* he wrote:

> In venturing to object to the opinions of Mr Hunter I do it with the greatest deference and respect; and if a sense of public duty did not make me feel it necessary to controvert what he has advanced relative to amputation in gunshot wounds, where it is not supported by fact, I would not willingly have avoided it; for it would have been more

grateful to confirm the opinions of the man whom all British surgeons must venerate as the founder of modern surgery, than to oppose them.[18]

Parts of many of his books were published in *The Lancet*, whose editor Thomas Wakley had become a personal friend after the libel episodes and remained so for many years. Guthrie repeatedly wrote letters to *The Lancet* on controversial matters of the time and always kept abreast of current thought. In the year of his death he wrote a letter describing four cases of wounds of the larynx and oesophagus, together with critical comments on their treatment.[19]

Perusal of his books shows that he had an extensive knowledge of previous work; he quotes extensively from the writings of English, European and American authors. His *Lancet* obituary said:

As an author and thinker he was most industrious and the vigorous and original powers of his mind will long impress the pathology and practice of surgery. In his meridian he was hardly more distinguished as a surgeon than as an anatomist. Forty years of peace could not dull the fire of the army surgeon.[20]

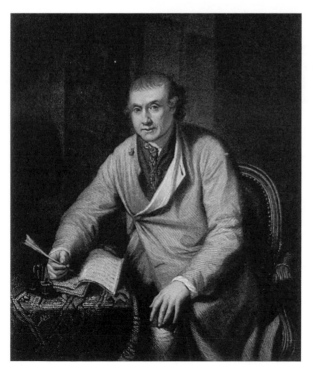

His first book, *Gun Shot Wounds of the Extremities*, described many of his contributions to war surgery made during the Peninsular War, and in a later edition and in subsequent articles in *The Lancet*, he had the satisfaction of seeing that these advances had been accepted by other writers, though in some cases they had been pirated many years later and advanced as something new.[17]

Two of his important later books were *Compound Fractures of the Extremities* in 1838, and *Wounds and Injuries of the Chest* in 1848. The former is mainly a personal

Figure 5.4 *John Hunter (1728–1793) as a younger man than is usually portrayed (reproduced with permission from the Wellcome Library, London)*

historical account of the Peninsular War and contains relatively little surgical input, though it does emphasize the considerable advantage of excision of an injured joint and consequent preservation of a limb, rather than amputation, an operation especially applicable to the arm; the book is fascinating to read and excerpts from it are included in Chapter 3. The latter is the first published book to be devoted entirely to this subject, and it also includes sections on medical diseases of the chest.

He had an empirical approach to any new treatment, which he advised surgeons to use until their own experience showed it to be incorrect.

Lectures

Guthrie's lectures were very popular, full of anecdotes and illustrative cases, often the patient himself being present. *The Lancet* published a criticism of lectures at London teaching hospitals in 1833 and said of Guthrie that his lectures were 'more oratorical in their communications and [that] their instructions spontaneously assume the formal garb of lectures'.[8] His considerable reputation as a lecturer caused 'some jealousy among his colleagues'.[8]

In 1851 he gave the Lettsomian Lecture on *Important Points in Surgery* at the Medical Society of London; unfortunately their *Transactions* for that year could not be located.[21]

His Hunterian Oration (reprinted in Chapter 14) was delivered at the Royal College of Surgeons in 1830, was said to be memorable and was delivered 'fluently and without notes'. 'It was a most marvellous effort', said one member of the audience, 'I shall not easily forget it'.[22] *The Lancet* was annoyed at its undoubted success and sneered at him as 'Orator Guthrie' but the remark fell on stony ground and was not accepted. 'I have heard many Hunterian Orations but I remember none more worthy of the name and more to the purpose than that of "Orator Guthrie".' The writer of these remarks had first met Guthrie at the Gerard School of Medicine, to which Guthrie gave lectures free of charge. He described his delivery as clear and with sound common sense. 'He invariably put on before lecturing a large check apron covering him entirely, and armlets of the same material – indeed he was always scrupulously clean in all he did and in his dress'[22,23] (Figures 5.5 and 5.6).

Guthrie, the man and his character

Guthrie was of only medium height, though heavily built, and was said to have very piercing eyes. He was highly intelligent

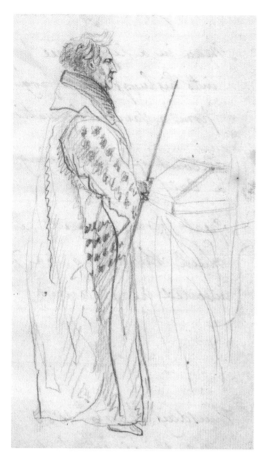

Figure 5.5 *Pencil sketch of Guthrie lecturing on emphysema May 6th 1830, 11th Lecture (note his mottled overall) (RCSSC P362) (see also Obituary, Chapter 9, p. 156) (reproduced with permission from the Royal College of Surgeons of England, London)*

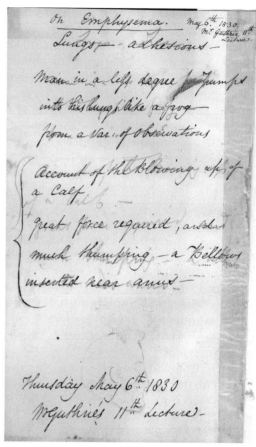

Figure 5.6 *Notes on Guthrie's lecture on emphysema: 'lungs – adhesions – man in a less degree – jumps into his lungs like a frog – from a variety of observations – account of the blowing up of a calf – great force required and much thumping – a bellows inserted near anus'. Thursday May 6th 1830. Mr Guthrie's 11th Lecture (reproduced with permission from the Royal College of Surgeons of England, London)*

and had a very practical and common sense approach to almost any problem, whether medical, non-medical or administrative, and this had led to his early appointment as sole medical officer in charge of his regiment in Canada. It was said that 'the adage of the accomplished operator may be truly applied to him – the lion heart, the eagle eye, the lady's hand'.[1] Furthermore, his operative technique was courageous and definite, as evidenced by his three dramatic operations after the battle of Waterloo (see Chapter 4, p. 66).

During the whole of his career Guthrie was extremely outspoken due to his honesty, sincerity and insistence on the truth, and fairness in all the decisions which he made. In the Preface to the 6th edition of the *Commentaries* he emphasized his wish to acknowledge the work of other surgeons and not to claim it as his own (see Chapter 11). He would often hurt other's feelings and more than once this led to serious conflict with the authorities. He was often somewhat brusque but nevertheless kind and generous, and he inspired a great sense of loyalty among his friends. He was extremely popular with both officers and men in his regiment, partly because of his professional skill and partly because of his garrulous personality. Some years after Guthrie had returned to civilian life the officers of his old regiment presented him with a silver loving cup suitably inscribed as a mark of the esteem in which he had been held.[1]

J. F. Clarke, for many years on the editorial staff of *The Lancet* and who knew him well, described him in 1874 as:

> Shrewd, quick, active and robust, always in good spirits, and most punctual in all his appointments. He was voluble to a fault. Everything that Guthrie said was to the point and practical but his fluency tempted him occasionally to say unwise things.[22]

During one of his lectures on cataract, an operation for which Guthrie was well known and excelled, he had said that before a surgeon could operate successfully, he must have 'put out a hatful of eyes'. This remark, off-the-cuff and to make a point, was taken literally by *The Lancet* which called the new Westminster Ophthalmic Hospital 'the blind manufactory'.[22] An action for libel was threatened but withdrawn at the last moment, the expense being paid by Guthrie.

He was an examiner to the Royal College of Surgeons from 1828 to 1856 and was greatly disliked and feared by students because of his severe and abrupt manner, so much so that many candidates would pay a fee to attend his lectures at Westminster Hospital in order *not* to have him as an examiner (a college examiner was not allowed to examine his own pupils).[24] Nevertheless it was said that he was always very fair and that he would never give a deciding vote against a candidate.[24] He abhorred the nepotism of the College of Surgeons and was successful in its elimination during his three Presidencies, but, nevertheless, he managed to establish his son Charles as his successor to the two hospitals to which he was attached, following his resignation from these institutions![6]

He was an independent and self-reliant character who had shaped his own career with little help from the surgical establishment and learnt his surgery in the field the hard way. He was a gadfly in every committee which he attended.[25]

He was fluent in French and Spanish and, during a lull in the fighting during the Peninsular War after the battle of Salamanca, he also became fluent in Portuguese.

J. F. Clarke wrote:

The more I saw of Guthrie the more I was impressed with the excellence of his heart and his real, good, honest nature. I was on terms of intimacy with him during the last few years of his life and had many opportunities of testing him. He was somewhat "off-hand" – brusque it may be said – some went so far as to think him offensive. But whatever the manner, the material was of the true metal – the "gold was the gold for all that". He was brilliant as an operator, shrewd in diagnosis, and though an uneducated man had all the natural attributes of a great surgeon.[22]

The remark about lack of education can be questioned, for his writings include many quotations in Latin and in French, and references to past classical literature; he clearly had considerable writing ability and must have had a good education.

The recent Oxford University study of army doctors in the 19th century described Guthrie as being a persistent social climber and a snob. Is this really a fair comment, for patronage in the 19th century had become essential to satisfy a natural ambition for an improved status in society?[26]

His private life was well described in *The Lancet*:

In private life his manner was most genial and kindly, and to those who knew him best he was ever most gentle and attaching. As a friend he was most kind and constant, always thoughtful of the welfare of those whose interests he had at heart. His friends will ever have cause to remember him with affectionate gratitude. There was something of Ireland, Scotland and England in his blood, and certainly he possessed a rich vein of the wit and humour of the first, the shrewd keenness and penetration of the second, mixed and timely tempered with the cosmopolitan sympathies of the third.[20]

His remarkable career is epitomized in the words of Pettigrew:

> Mr Guthrie's life has been one of unwearied activity and
> indefatigable research. He has laboriously studied to learn
> and improve the profession of which he is an ornament. In
> his character as a lecturer he is distinguished by peculiar
> earnestness, precision and vivacity. He has a great command
> of language and mixes in a most agreeable manner personal
> anecdotes and descriptions with the relation of his cases,
> so that they cannot fail to make a strong impression on his
> hearers. Mr Guthrie indeed appears to be as much a soldier
> as a surgeon; and the advantages likely to arise from the
> possession of such combined qualities need not be pointed
> out. In his discourses and his writings he has never omitted
> any opportunity of asserting the high importance of
> anatomical knowledge to the successful cultivation of
> surgical science. In proportion to the eagerness displayed
> by any individual for the acquisition of professional
> knowledge will always be found a desire to advance the
> interests and dignity of the profession.[27]

The Lancet eulogy in 1856, immediately following his death, is
equally laudable, though this is perhaps expected in view of the
journal's editor who presumably wrote or commissioned it:

> His early entrance into the profession; his precocious
> distinction as an army surgeon; his eminent services in the
> Peninsular War, of which he afterwards became the surgical
> historian; his success as the leading surgeon in this great
> metropolis for upwards of a quarter of a century; his triple
> Presidency of the College which he joined as boy of sixteen,
> are universally known to the medical public. Not so well
> known are the generous virtues and rare qualities of mind
> and heart which graced his private life, and the remem-
> brance of which give at once poignancy and consolation
> to those who mourn him most deeply.[20]

Was he a showman at heart?

Perhaps he was, as many surgeons have been in the past, and he
certainly gave this impression during his lectures and some of
his operations – the large check apron already mentioned whilst
lecturing suggest this. He also preferred manual compression of
the axillary or femoral artery rather than the use of a tourniquet
during an amputation of an arm or leg, and on more than one
occasion he had released the pressure on the main artery to

allow the blood to spurt out over the onlookers if they had irritated him or approached too close (see Chapter 3, p. 49).

His compassionate nature

Despite his brusqueness and his quick tongue, Guthrie (Figure 5.7) was a humane surgeon, compassionate, sympathetic and understanding of others, and this was well shown by his vivid description of a hospital ward after the battle of Salamanca in the Peninsular campaign (see Chapter 2, p. 23) and his statement that he found his army medical work 'grim in the extreme, alleviated only by the heroism of the suffering soldiers'.[28] He also expressed his feelings in Aphorism 144 in the *Commentaries*:

> War is an agreeable occupation, trade or professional employment for the few only, not for the many; and particularly not for the poor when they have the misfortune to have their limbs broken by musket-shot. ... The nation at large shall be impressed with the idea that no expense, no trouble ought to be spared to procure for their soldiers so unhappily injured the utmost comfort and accommodation that can be procured for them as well as the best surgical assistance. Many a gallant soldier lost his life from the want of that proper attendance and care alluded to; many a desolate and unhappy mother mourned the loss of a son she need not have mourned for under happier circumstances and who might have been the support, the happiness of her declining years. Yet England calls herself the most humane as well as the greatest nation upon earth; she claims to be the most civilised and she may be so ... but she could not on many occasions have been more careless or less compassionate. I have endeavoured to impress the injustice, the carelessness of the treatment of the wounded soldiers

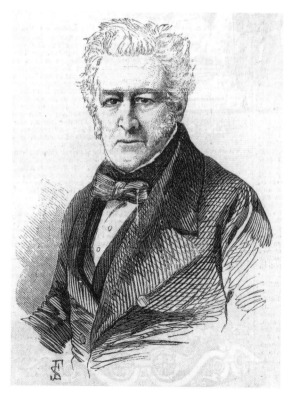

Figure 5.7 *Pen drawing of Guthrie from a daguerrotype by Mayall (reproduced with permission from the Wellcome Library)*

of the royal army of Great Britain. My remonstrations have hitherto been in great part useless. ... A public enquiry can alone cause this grievance to be redressed. Old habits are not to be overcome but by public opinion.[29]

The present lack of proper protection for army personnel in Afghanistan is very similar to the sentiments expressed by Guthrie 150 years ago. *Plus ça change, plus c'est la même chose.*

His modesty, humility and consideration for others

Perhaps surprisingly he was often remarkably modest: 'I am a man without a wish – without desire – for anything which belongs to this world,' he wrote in the Preface to *Wounds and Injuries of the Chest.*[30] Furthermore, he had been asked why he had presumed to 'obtrude his opinions on anyone, much more on the great Civil authorities of this country who do not desire them?'

> The answer is simple. There is no one who ought to understand the subject so well, although there are many persons who do understand it better. It has been enquired what place I am seeking to obtain? The answer is more simple still. ... I seek a place in which I and all the authorities which I have ventured to address shall one day stand before Him by whose all-seeing eye our innermost thoughts will be laid bare, and when I earnestly pray that my endeavours on behalf of the helpless may be favourably judged.[30]

This epitomizes his philosophy, his attitude to his profession and his dedication to military surgery throughout his life. He then went on to write:

> Follow implicitly the precepts I have laid down until you have reason, from your own observation or from that of others, to doubt. A little further experience will then enable you to confirm what I have said or to lay down, in turn, other principles which, whilst they supersede mine, may be of more service to mankind.[31]

These precepts were very different from those which had prevailed before the Peninsular War.

After Waterloo Guthrie treated many battle casualties who had been returned to England and in his lectures he was often critical of their previous treatment, but he seldom divulged the names of those who had treated them previously:

> Whenever I have not approved of the practice pursued by my contemporaries I have rarely named the surgeon in charge of it. I want merely the fact for the benefit of science, not the inculpation of an individual.[32]

Request for appointment as Serjeant Surgeon

The office of Serjeant Surgeon is one of great antiquity and the principal duty of the recipient was to attend the monarch during his military activities. An appointment to this prestigious position had previously been supported privately and publicly by the Dukes of York and Wellington, and also by Lords Hill and Vivian, respectively Commander-in-Chief and Master General of the British Army. A vacancy for this appointment had arisen following the death of Sir Astley Cooper in 1841 and Guthrie wished his name to be put forward on the grounds of his public service during the Peninsular War. He wrote to Lord Peel requesting his support and said:

> I served during the Peninsular War, from the first battle to the last, was chief on the field on several occasions, and had larger and more important charges than any other officer save the two successive heads of the Department, Dr Franck and Sir James McGrigor. During this period I was enabled by continual labours under constant opportunity to form those opinions, establish those principles, and lay down those precepts which overturned all those that preceded them.
>
> After the battle of Waterloo, when the greatest distress was impending from the want of efficient surgeons, I went to Brussels and carried into execution during five weeks those precepts which otherwise might have been neglected. … I had the good fortune to perform operations which had not been done before, or had not succeeded in either the foreign or the British armies or in private life. On my return to London I willingly took charge (without pay) in the York Hospital, Chelsea of the worst cases which came from Waterloo, and this labour which I continued for years enabled me to perfect the observations I had previously made, and I have willingly taught them gratuitously to the officers of the public service.

It was on this occasion that His Royal Highness the late Duke of York ... was pleased to express his approbation of my services and to promise me his favour with the view of obtaining the office I now solicit. The office of third Serjeant Surgeon would give me neither precedence nor emolument, but it would show to the public, especially to foreigners, that to have served under the Medical Department of the Army with some distinction was considered in England as well as abroad, a source of merit deserving approbation.[33]

Guthrie's application was not successful.

Notes and references

1. Biographical sketch. *Lancet* 1850; **1**: 733–4.
2. Ackroyd M, Brockliss L, Moss M, Retford K, Stevenson J. *Advancing with the Army.* Oxford: Oxford University Press, 2007, p. 321.
3. Royal College of Surgeons of England. *Tract* 1827; **138**(9).
4. Spencer WG. *Westminster Hospital.* London: Glaisler, 1924, p. 104.
5. Langdon-Davies J. *Westminster Hospital.* London: Murray, 1952, p. 110, 188.
6. Yearsley PM. George James Guthrie. *Westminster Hosp J* 1892; 1–8. (A lecture to the Guthrie Society on 9th June 1892.)
7. Grimsdale H. George James Guthrie FRS. *Br J Ophthalmol* 1919; **3**: 144–52.
8. Humble JG, Hansell P. *Westminster Hospital 1716–1974,* 2nd edn. London: Pitman, 1974, pp. 57–8.
9. *Proc R Soc* 1856–7; **8**: 273. Cited in ref. 2, p. 297.
10. Guthrie GJ. *Commentaries on the Surgery of the War,* 5th edn. London: Renshaw, 1853, Lecture 1, p. 5, 7.
11. Ballance CA. *J R Army Med Corp* 1917; **29**: 357–74.
12. Op. cit. ref. 2, p. 55.
13. Cule JH. Some observations of George Guthrie on gunshot wounds of the thigh during the Crimean War. *J R Soc Med* 1991; **84**: 675–7.
14. Obituary. *Association Medical Journal* 1856: 389, 394 (precursor of *British Medical Journal*).
15. Porter JH. *The Surgeon's Pocket Book.* London: Griffin, 1875.

16. Op. cit. ref. 10. 6th edn. p. 260.

17. Pettigrew TJ. *Biographical Memoirs of Physicians and Surgeons*. London: Whittaker, 1840, p. 11, 13, 18 and 22.

18. Guthrie GJ. Preface. In: *A Treatise on Gun Shot Wounds of the Extremities*. Burgess and Hill, 1815, pp. v–vi.

19. Guthrie GJ. Cases in military surgery occurring in the Crimea. *Lancet* 1856; **1**: 65–7.

20. Obituary. *Lancet* 1856: **1**: 519–20.

21. Could not be located at the British Library, Medical Society of London, Royal College of Surgeons of England, Royal Society of Medicine Library or Wellcome Library.

22. Clarke JF. *Autobiographical Recollections of the Medical Profession*. London: Churchill, 1874, pp. 259–61, 293. J.F. Clarke had for many years been on the editorial staff of *The Lancet*.

23. Op. cit. ref. 2, p. 248.

24. Heath C. Guthrie and the old hospital. *Broadway* March 1962; **R18**, No. 234: 218.

25. Williams DI. *R Coll Surg Engl Bull* 1996; **78**: 285.

26. Op. cit. ref. 2, p. 267.

27. Op. cit. ref. 17, p. 21.

28. Laffin J. *Surgeons in the Field*. London: Dent, 1970, p. 86.

29. Op. cit. ref. 10, p. 140.

30. Guthrie GJ. Preface. In: *Wounds and Injuries of the Chest*. London: Renshaw, 1848, p. 3.

31. Op. cit. ref. 29, p. 1 (Preface).

32. Guthrie GJ. *Wounds and Injuries of the Arteries*. London: Churchill, 1830, p. 61.

33. British Library. Additional MSS 40477, folio 27. Memorial 1841. Peel papers. (This letter was written by hand and signed by G.J. Guthrie.)

CHAPTER 6

Presidency of the Royal College of Surgeons of England

G eorge Guthrie became a Member of Council of the Royal College of Surgeons in London (later of England) in 1824 when aged 39, a younger age than anyone previously, and he immediately became actively involved in its administration during one of the most crucial and turbulent periods in its history. In May 1824 an extraordinary resolution for membership of Council had been proposed which was clearly directed towards Guthrie, presumably by a faction of Council members who did not wish him to be elected:

> In the event of the election of a person to be a member of Council who shall be a surgeon of any institution for the special treatment of diseases of the eye or ear, he be informed he will be expected to resign such institution as soon as his resignation can be effected.[1]

Nevertheless he was elected to Council the following month as the resolution was clearly unfair and unenforceable, for Guthrie had founded the Westminster Ophthalmic Hospital in 1816, was well-known as an eye surgeon and, moreover, remained on the staff of this hospital until his resignation in 1838. During the next 20 years he was five times Vice-President and three times President of the College – in 1833, in 1841 and finally in 1854.

Until he was elected to Council, he and other members of the College had been obliged to enter the College by the back door in Portugal Street ('an invidious and offensive distinction')[2] rather than by the front door in Lincoln's Inn Fields (Figure 6.1), and to 'place themselves outside a bar erected for the preservation of the places of the favoured and to such other little indignitories as were at that time supposed to be necessary to inflict on the many, to do honour to the few'.[2] It was several years before Guthrie was able to persuade Council to amend this injustice; the bar was eventually removed and every member was then allowed to enter by the front door on production of evidence of identity to the College porter. Furthermore, he insisted that increased access to the Hunterian Museum be permitted; previously, the times of entry had been severely restricted.

Election to Council

Just as his appointment to the Westminster Hospital revolutionized its organization,[3] so must have been the effect on the College of Surgeons after his appointment to Council, though his three times Presidency showed how effective he must have been and how well his leadership was accepted. On College Council he continually strove to promote justice and openness in its administration and to abolish nepotism in College appointments. He did much to reform the administration of the College and in this he was ably supported by the energetic Thomas Wakley, an influential member of the College who had founded *The Lancet* in 1823 to 'report medical lectures and to expose nepotism in hospital appointments'.[4] Wakley became a Member of Parliament in 1835 and had been an early and prominent

Figure 6.1 *The Royal College of Surgeons in London in 1813 (reproduced with permission from the Royal College of Surgeons of England, London)*

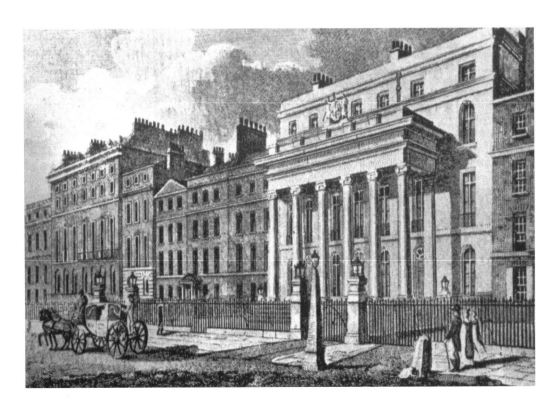

critic of College affairs. Guthrie 'contended that the affairs of the College of Surgeons required no secrecy but that they should be founded on strict equity and justice; that he was ready at all times to submit his own views to the investigation of the profession, on whose good sense and justice he relied with the most perfect confidence'.[2]

Immediately after his election to Council Guthrie familiarized himself with all the College papers, 'both ancient and modern', and he then 'addressed the Council on the inconveniences occasioned by their restrictions which caused so much dissatisfaction to their members'.[2] That a councillor of only one year's standing should request that these restrictions be altered surprised everyone. He explained that they were acting illegally, were in flagrant violation of the College Charter and were liable to censure in the Court of the King's Bench as well as possible forfeiture of the College Charter itself. 'The affairs of the College of Surgeons', he said, 'should be conducted like the affairs of the nation. How can the constituency judge of their worthiness when their speeches, their votes, their acts are, as at present, secret?'[2] Guthrie tabled many proposals for reform which were all referred to the standing Council of the College, which eventually agreed that Guthrie was correct in most of his suggestions; and thenceforth all executive decisions were referred to Council rather than being decided secretly behind closed doors.[2] In all this he had been ably supported and encouraged by Keate and Vincent, both senior members of Council.

Mr Carpue, under whom he had worked at York Hospital and who had reconstructed a nose on two patients in 1814 using a skin graft turned down from the forehead (as had been done by early Hindu surgeons), had established a private school of anatomy in Dean Street. He was an influential member of Council and had become head of the radicals in the College. He said to Guthrie after one of his proposals had been accepted against the wishes of some other senior members of Council: 'My good fellow, you have saved your College but you have ruined yourself. The surgeon apothecaries will never patronise you'.[5] Guthrie replied: 'My dear Mr Carpue, they never have; I cannot, therefore lose what I have never had'. Guthrie said that he had always done them more than justice; he could not help them being ungrateful, but this would not prevent him continuing to serve them.[6] The surgeon apothecaries were members of the College who mainly practised surgery, as opposed to the large number of other members who practised physic (medicine) as well. The future wide scope of operative surgery had not yet been appreciated – this did not occur until the mid-19th century with the introduction of anaesthesia.[7]

During the early years of the newly formed College, new members were elected by the present Council members themselves – a self-perpetuating body whose members held office for life and who resisted change; a system which was clearly unfair. The younger members thought that Council should be chosen from the whole College membership. However, this was complicated by the fact that some members did not confine themselves to pure surgery. At a Select Committee in 1834 Guthrie was asked, 'Was not a large part of Abernethy's [who had been President in 1826] practice of a medical kind?', to which he replied, 'So is my own: and so is every surgeon in London'.[8]

Liberal Party in College Council

The Lancet obituary aptly stated:

> In all that related to medical policy Mr Guthrie was staunchly liberal. He was long the leader of the Liberal Party in the Council of the College of Surgeons, and the main author and promoter of almost every liberal measure which has marked the progress of the College in late years. At the same time he was devoted to the true interests of the College which he believed to be the greatest medical institution in the country. One of the last interests for which he strove in the Council was the institution of an examination in preliminary general education for students intending to pass the College diploma examination.[9]

He continued to urge for a reform of the Charter of 1843, which his obituary in *The Lancet* (whose editor was Wakley, Guthrie's close friend) had described as obnoxious (see Chapter 9, p. 145). Guthrie was very much a self-made man who had established himself as an eminent surgeon during his military service in Portugal, Spain and at Waterloo, and he resented the 'closed shop' attitude of the London teaching hospitals' staff, who were chosen from their own apprentices and relatives, and who dominated College affairs.[7]

Reform of College Charter

The original Charter granted by Charles I to the Barber Surgeons Company of London in 1629 remained in force for almost 200 years. When the Royal College of Surgeons in London was founded in 1800 this Charter was considered to be unsatisfactory; a further revision was begun in 1832 and was only reluctantly accepted 13 years later in 1843, 10 years after

Guthrie's first Presidency. It was at that time, too, that the name was changed to the Royal College of Surgeons of England. The early 19th century had been a time of great change, as was noted in the introduction to the first *Medical Directory* in 1847, when it was recognized that the profession was becoming divided into those in general practice and those in consulting practice. The College rightly wished to introduce a Fellowship examination to recognize those surgeons who were fully trained to a high standard.

Soon after its foundation the College proposed its own Bill to regulate the training of surgeons and tried to gain control of all surgery in Great Britain and Ireland, but, not surprisingly, the older Scottish and Irish Surgical Colleges objected. Finally in 1832 a committee of younger surgeons was formed under the chairmanship of a liberal-minded senior member of Council, Sir Astley Cooper, 'to consider the present state of the College'. Its first report a year later showed that 'a new spirit had arisen within the Council, unquestionably through the influence of the younger men, but supported by several of their seniors'.[10] This committee had included George Guthrie. The suggested Charter proposed an end to life membership for Council members, a review of medical education and the establishment of a Fellowship of the College by examination, with future members of Council being elected by the Fellows.

Membership of the College Council and of the College

Guthrie had adamantly opposed life membership for Council members and in this he had been supported by Wakley, who said that 'the whole mismanagement of the College results from the manner in which the Council and Court of Examiners elect each other'. At a committee meeting in 1834, one year after Guthrie had become President, he was asked: 'The persons once elected to Council remain so for life?' Guthrie replied: 'They do; that is a point that needs alteration'.[11]

In 1815 the Apothecaries Act had raised the standard of medical education and this stimulated the College to abolish the system of surgical apprenticeship and to introduce a set curriculum. Regulations for the membership of the College were changed and, amongst other proposals, it was considered that the period of study be reduced from six to five years, for (they said) 'the greater part of this time is passed in an apothecary's shop, where little is learned beyond the business of the chemist and druggist'.[12] In fact, it was thought that three years' intensive study would be sufficient.

Examination for membership of the College

In 1834 the procedure to be followed by a candidate for examination for membership was well described by Guthrie:

> When a gentleman believes that he has qualified himself as far as he is required by the printed regulations he produces his certificates to the secretary; who desires him to fix his own time for the examination. The two junior examiners look over the certificates. The President takes the chair and the members of the Court assemble. The candidate is introduced and placed at the bottom of a horse-shoe table *[Figure 6.2]*. The President usually directs that one member shall examine him. It is common for the person sitting next to that member to take a share and if any misunderstanding arises he assists the examiner. At the same time the whole Court interferes whenever it pleases, asking such questions as any examiner may think proper. The President then asks whether any gentlemen would wish to examine the candidate further. The candidate is then desired to withdraw and the gentleman who examined is called upon to state whether he considers the candidate qualified or not. If he is satisfied he expresses his opinion to that effect. If that is not seconded it is then put to the vote.[13]

Figure 6.2 *The examination of young surgeons. George Cruikshank lampoons the licence proceedings in 1811 (reproduced with permission from the Royal College of Surgeons of England, London)*

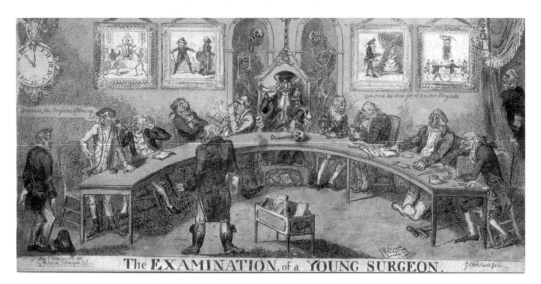

A higher surgical examination leading to Fellowship

A higher surgical examination was also suggested, at first to be limited to lecturers in anatomy, physiology and surgery. This was clearly impracticable. Guthrie wished to make this qualification open to all members of the College 'who were desirous of obtaining this honour', who were also to be chosen 'by nomination of those surgeons and teachers of recognised hospitals whom the Council should select and partly by examination, which should be open to all members of not less than five years' standing and at least 25 years of age'.[14] It seemed that Guthrie was against Fellowship by examination only, which would have been the only way to distinguish a fully trained consultant surgeon from a general practitioner with a special interest, who would carry out the occasional operation when required. He did not seem to appreciate how operative surgery would develop in the future or how general practitioners and consultants would eventually become separate groups within the profession.[7]

The new Charter

The new Charter was finally agreed by Council in 1843 and the same year was passed by Parliament, which gratuitously also suggested that in future the College should be known as the Royal College of Surgeons of England.[15] The Charter created several hundred Fellows, mainly but not exclusively from London, to be nominated by Council and a year later the remainder would be selected by examination. Life tenure of Council was abolished and Council members were to be elected for a limited number of years by the College membership. Unfortunately the new Charter excluded from nomination for Fellowship many established surgeons in the armed forces and the East India Company; only five nominations were from the army and navy as Council had little information about the remainder.[16]

Opposition to the new Charter

Not surprisingly Guthrie and also Wakley were bitterly opposed to the exclusion of the armed forces and some other details of the new Charter. Guthrie felt so strongly about this that he presented his own individual petition of protest to the House of Commons. 'He stood alone in opposition to it ... declaring that its sole merit was its remarkable abstinence from anything like law, equity or justice'.[17]

Extracts from 'the petition of Mr Guthrie, the celebrated army surgeon', reported in *The Times* on 7th July 1844, a year after its acceptance by the College, include:

> He *[Guthrie]* considers several of the provisions of the said Charter to be illiberal, exclusive and unjust. That, independently of its placing a bar on the poor man, preventing in many cases his obtaining by his own exertions such places of honour as there may be in the profession of surgery, it offers unnecessary advantages to the richer student in the attainment of these offices who may not possess half his ability, his perseverance or his knowledge, it presses with peculiar severity on the officers of the public service, nearly the whole of whom are deprived by it of those privileges they hitherto enjoyed, in common with their surgical brethren of equal standing in civil life; whilst they will also be deprived in future of the hope of succeeding to these offices of honour or profit, whatever may be their ability, or the pre-eminence they may have acquired in the service of their country.

He then went on to say that he himself, who had twice been President of the College, could not have been elected to this office under the proposed rules of the Charter. Furthermore, many surgeons who had served in the armed forces or the East India Company would now find themselves omitted 'from the rights and privileges they have hitherto enjoyed'. He believed 'that the evil which has been committed has been unintentional and that it can be remedied by a supplement to the said Charter'.[18]

Wakley was of the same opinion and in an outspoken editorial in the influential *The Lancet* on 7th October 1843 said that 'the profession will hear with the utmost astonishment and indignation and disgust the grant of a new Charter to the College of Surgeons of London: that institution which of all others has been the most denounced for its unjust and atrocious conduct towards the members of its own body'.[19] He later wrote in *The Lancet*, 'a more mischievous, a more iniquitous Charter never was honoured with the sign manual of the Crown'.[17] The College had also received demands from the senior officers in the army (Sir James McGrigor) and the navy (Sir William Burnett) requesting that a large number of their officers (200 from the navy alone) be granted Fellowship. This could not be accepted as it would have inevitably led to the management of the College being dominated by the armed forces.[20] The outcome of this opposition to the new Charter, which had been very much orchestrated by Thomas Wakley and his College Council supporter George Guthrie, was that one year later in 1844 a new list of 242 nominations for Fellowship was produced and this included 13 from the army, 21 from the navy and 11 from the East India Company. This compromise was reluctantly accepted and Guthrie's main objection to the Charter was satisfied.

In 1843 Guthrie had also surprisingly proposed that all members of the College of 20 years' standing be admitted as Fellows, a move which would have seriously undermined the reputation of the Fellowship, the aim of which was to set a minimum standard for recognition as a competent surgeon. Wisely this was not approved by Council.

College Professor of Anatomy and Surgery

During his Presidencies Guthrie (Figure 6.3) was College Professor of Anatomy and Surgery for five years and he gave a series of lectures which were always well attended. They were:

1. *On the Anatomy and Diseases of the Arterial System,* 'in which he developed his views on the treatment of wounded arteries, in opposition to the opinions then commonly entertained', in particular his advocacy of ligation of *both* ends of an injured artery, a very important contribution (see Chapter 15).
2. *On the Anatomy and Diseases of the Eye* (see Chapter 13).
3. *On Some Points in the Anatomy and Treatment of Hernia,* 'in which he was the first to show the impropriety and danger of the practice of administering active purgatives after the operation'.
4. *On the Anatomy and Diseases of the Urinary and Sexual Organs,* 'demonstrating some points unobserved in the structure of the bladder, and also a muscle of the urethra, distinct from those previously described', which sometimes is named after him, as well as named *'constrictor urethrae'* (see Chapter 18).
5. *On the Anatomy of the Brain and on Injuries of the Head,* in which he showed that the so-called more modern improvements in treatment had been successfully practised during the latter part of the Peninsular War.[2]

During his time as Professor he founded scholarships in anatomy (human and comparative) and natural history, for three years, at £100 per annum (£6560 in 2006), and assistant surgeoncies in the army and navy to deserving students at the end of each term.[21]

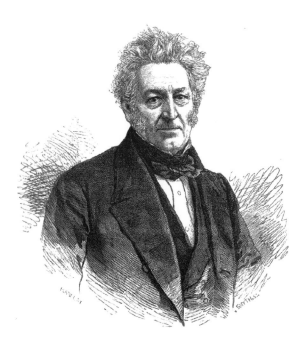

Figure 6.3 *Pen drawing of Guthrie (reproduced with permission from* The Lancet*)*

Reform of military surgery

In the early 19th century there was no organized medical corps and each medical officer wore the uniform of the regiment to which he was attached. Furthermore there were also many 'Apothecaries to the Forces', who in civil life had been chemists. There had been a desperate need to improve the provision of an army medical service and Guthrie was influential in trying to effect change. Even at the time of the Crimean War (1853–6), the so-called Medical Staff Corps (successor to the 'Apothecaries to the Forces') was composed of men of poor education, who had received no special training and who did not have their own officers. 'The lower situations were held by men, who being nearly precluded from all hope of advancement, were frequently careless of improvement' (see also Guthrie's 'Dedication to the Duke of York' in Chapter 10, p. 161). However, in 1857, one year after Guthrie's death, an Army Hospital Corps was established of specially trained men with non-medical officers. This was a major improvement and led to the inauguration of the Royal Army Medical Corps by Queen Victoria in 1898.[22] Guthrie's dream of a fully trained medical corps had at long last been fulfilled.

In the early 19th century the quality of military surgery was low, as also were the qualifications and standards of the surgeons themselves. As Guthrie testified to the 1840 Royal Commission on Promotion in the Army and Navy:

> The whole service was still treated in a contemptuous and humiliating manner. I have seen a Staff-Surgeon in charge of many hundred wounded brush his shoes, clean his own horse and then go out to do many of the most delicate operations in surgery.[23]

And furthermore the army surgeon was:

The most neglected officer in the service. It is only to the surgeons of the army that promotion or honours or pension are considered unnecessary and are absolutely refused. Medical officers are human beings, subject to the same influences, feelings and passions as other men. They should have held out to them at all times the same or similar inducements to good conduct, to exertion and to emulation in their profession found necessary and proper for the services of the army at large.[23]

During his time on Council Guthrie continued to press for an improved image and status for army surgeons, partly by his own influence and partly by persuasion of his colleagues to press for effective action. He also wrote frequently to *The Lancet* on this subject. He had helped to improve the quality of the army surgical service by sending a copy of his *Commentaries* at his own expense to each regiment in the British army, so that its surgeons were aware of the correct management of war injuries. He campaigned, though unsuccessfully, for a Chair of Military Surgery along the lines of that in Edinburgh (then the centre of British medical learning), which had been established in 1803, as had one later in Dublin in 1851.[22]

Most of the Preface to *Wounds and Injuries of the Chest,* published in 1840, is devoted to reform of the army medical service, and even in his 60s, when he had left Council, he continued to campaign for this. After his death a School of Military Surgery was finally established at Fort Pitt, Chatham in 1860,[24] and later transferred to Netley Hospital, Southampton.

Anatomy Act 1832

Guthrie was very much involved with the passing of the Anatomy Act in 1832, which put an end to the activities of the 'resurrectionists' or bodysnatchers, who had robbed recent graves in Dublin, Edinburgh and London in order to sell bodies for dissection. Until this time very few bodies could be obtained legitimately and there was little opportunity for medical students to dissect a human body. The few demonstrations were surrounded by an aura of suspicion and the strong iron railings still found in some churchyards are a reminder of those days. An earlier Bill to regulate the study of anatomy had been rejected by Parliament. A corpse (murdered or disinterred) could be sold for £10 (£656 in 2006) and after a few days it was not possible to tell 'under what circumstances the body was deprived of life'.[25] In 1831 one of the corpses obtained in London 'had been taken to King's College, within a stone's throw of the College', and an attempt had been made to sell the body to the Professor of Anatomy. An emergency meeting of Council was held 'in consequence of the fearful events which have lately, for a second time, been brought to light'. Representation was made to Parliament and Guthrie wrote a 3500-word letter to Lord Althorp for distribution to Members of Parliament and the House of Lords providing the arguments for such a Bill to enable an adequate supply of cadavers for dissection (Figure 6.4). He described five ways in which 'a significant supply of dead bodies could be obtained'[25] and this assisted the passing of the Anatomy Act the same year. An adequate legal supply of human cadavers was now possible and the educational requirements of the College were facilitated.

Remuneration of Poor-Law surgeons

Guthrie took an active part in trying to change the law regulating the management of the sick poor and persuaded Council to address the Minister on this subject. This was not successful and so Guthrie himself approached the Secretary of State, who at first agreed to a £100 000 improvement scheme but then retracted the offer. The intention had been to improve the pay of the Poor-Law surgeons and to provide proper remuneration for each patient that they saw, both of which Guthrie had thought to be inadequate. Furthermore, they were expected to provide medicines free.[7] Unfortunately the proposal was rejected by Parliament, despite the support of Thomas Wakley and the influential *The Lancet*. However, Guthrie was successful later in persuading the Poor-Law Board to raise the standard of their medical officers and improve their pay.[9]

College Museum and Library in 1842

When Guthrie was President for the second time in 1842–3 a major change in the affairs

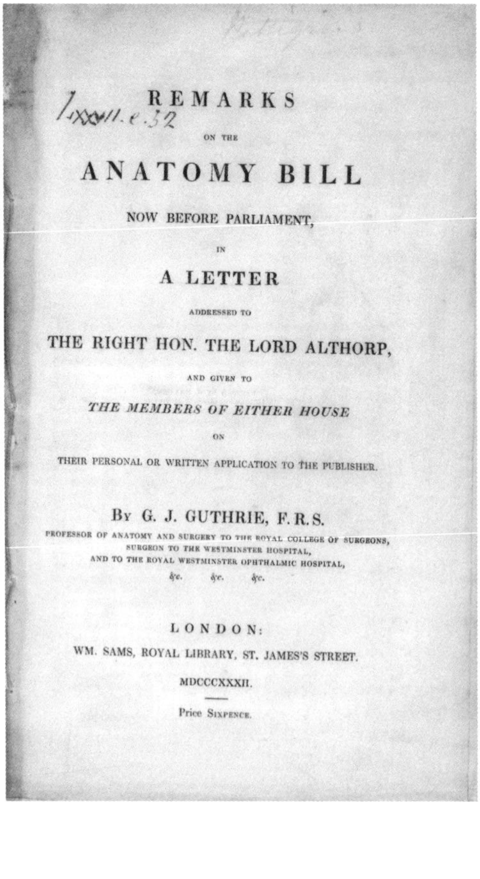

REMARKS

ON THE

ANATOMY BILL

NOW BEFORE PARLIAMENT,

IN

A LETTER

ADDRESSED TO

THE RIGHT HON. THE LORD ALTHORP,

AND GIVEN TO

THE MEMBERS OF EITHER HOUSE

ON

THEIR PERSONAL OR WRITTEN APPLICATION TO THE PUBLISHER.

BY G. J. GUTHRIE, F.R.S.

PROFESSOR OF ANATOMY AND SURGERY TO THE ROYAL COLLEGE OF SURGEONS, SURGEON TO THE WESTMINSTER HOSPITAL, AND TO THE ROYAL WESTMINSTER OPHTHALMIC HOSPITAL, &c. &c. &c.

LONDON:

WM. SAMS, ROYAL LIBRARY, ST. JAMES'S STREET.

MDCCCXXXII.

Price SIXPENCE.

Figure 6.4 *Three and a half thousand word letter concerning the Anatomy Bill to Lord Althorp (reproduced with permission from the Wellcome Library, London)* of the College was made – the contents of the museum were carefully assessed and 'everything objectionable or useless was destroyed'.[6] The public days were increased from three to four each week, 'every clean and decently dressed person had the right to ask for permission from the secretary' to visit the museum, and the remaining two days were allocated to special college students. Access to library facilities was also greatly improved.

Changes in regulations for the College Diploma in 1839

In 1839 Guthrie proposed the formation of a Court of Examiners in Midwifery, the incorporation of 'physic' into the examination, that the course of hospital study be increased from two to three years and that the minimum age for application for membership be reduced from 22 to 21. These proposals were accepted, though not without much opposition.[6] Prior to this 'he had never voted for the rejection of any candidate for the Diploma of the College on the ground that the examination was more searching than the course warranted'.[6]

Guthrie's involvement in politics whilst President of the Royal College of Surgeons of England – a summary

Guthrie's extensive involvement in politics, both medical and non-medical, was remarkable for someone who also had an active, extensive and successful surgical career (Figure 6.5). During his three Presidencies in 1833, 1841 and 1854 (this last in his 69th year), he revolutionized the College of Surgeons, which until this time had been governed by a self-perpetuating Council whose members were elected for life; it was obvious that this was bad for the College and required urgent change. He was prominent in the reform of the original Charter granted to the Barber–Surgeons and this led to rationalization of the training of surgeons by the introduction of a membership examination and also a higher Fellowship degree to confirm surgical competence. The new Charter had its faults but its introduction was a great achievement.

Until the mid-19th century the provision of medical care to the army had been poor and throughout his life Guthrie continued to press for the formation of a properly trained medical corps.

Figure 6.5 *This is the only known profile of Guthrie. It was drawn in 1890 and was based on a crayon portrait (which can not now be traced) by Count D'Orsay in the Westminster Hospital. The framed portrait had been presented to the Guthrie Society of the Westminster Hospital by Mr P. Macleod Yearsley, a surgeon and a historian, on 18th March 1890, who gave a lecture on Guthrie to the Society on 9th June 1892. It was rescued from a rubbish skip at the time of closure of the Westminster Hospital in the 1990s by a member of the engineering department, Mr Sidney Wright, who presented it to the author. The portrait is also reproduced in the* 2nd edition of Westminster Hospital 1716-1974 *by Humble JG and Hansell P., 1974 on p. 75.*

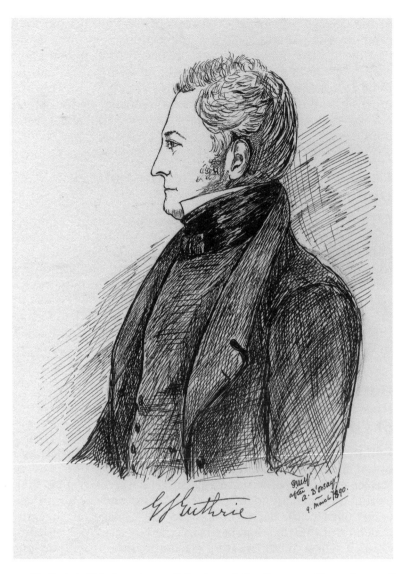

Guthrie's third major political contribution was the reform of the Anatomy Act in 1832, whereby the activities of the 'resurrectionists' were abolished and a legal supply of human bodies for study and research was made possible.

Many of the privileges now enjoyed by members and fellows of the College emanate from the major reforms which George Guthrie established during his Presidencies in the early 19th century.

Notes and references

1. Cope Z. *The Royal College of Surgeons of England*. London: Blunt, 1959, pp. 58, 72–3.

2. Biographical sketch. *Lancet* 1850; **1**: 735.

3. Humble JG, Hansell P. *Westminster Hospital 1716–1974*, 2nd edn. London: Pitman, 1974.

4. Obituary. Wakley. *Dictionary of National Biography* 1890; **23**: 375–6.

5. In about 1813 the surgeons and apothecaries united and called themselves 'The Society of Apothecaries and Surgeon–Apothecaries'. Op. cit. ref. 1, p. 36.

6. Op. cit. ref. 2, pp. 735–6.

7. Personal communication, Williams DI, 2007.

8. Op. cit. ref. 1, p. 58.

9. Obituary. *Lancet* 1856; **1**: 520.

10. Op. cit. ref. 1, p. 52.

11. Op. cit. ref. 1, p. 46.

12. Op. cit. ref. 1, p. 53.

13. Op. cit. ref. 1, p. 136.

14. Op. cit. ref. 1, pp. 64–5.

15. Op. cit. ref. 1, pp. 68–9.

16. Williams DI. *Ann R Coll Surg Engl (Suppl)* 1996; **78**: 283–8.

17. Op. cit. ref. 1, pp. 70–1.

18. *The Times* 27 July 1844, Issue 18673, p. 8, Col. G.

19. *Lancet* 1843; **1**: 23. Also op. cit. ref. 1, p. 736.

20. Op. cit. ref. 1, p. 73.

21. Pettigrew TJ. *Biographical Memoirs of Physicians and Surgeons*. London: Whittaker, 1840, p. 10.

22. Guthrie D. *A History of Medicine*. London: Nelson, 1945, pp. 344–7. The Dublin Chair was abolished in 1860 (see Widdess JDH. *The Royal College of Surgeons of Ireland 1784–1984*. Dublin: Royal College of Surgeons in Ireland, 1984).

23. Parliamentary Report on Promotion in the Army and Navy (1840), pp. 202–3, 278 (from Guthrie's evidence given on 19th March 1839). Cited by Ackroyd et al., ref. 24, p. 55.

24. Ackroyd M, Brockliss R, Moss M, Retford K, Stevenson J. *Advancing with the Army*. Oxford: Oxford University Press, 2006, p. 43.

25. Remarks on the Anatomy Bill. A letter to Lord Althorp, 1832.

CHAPTER 7

Later years and family

Throughout Guthrie's life his prime interest was military surgery, even after he had retired from his London practice. His great work, the *Commentaries*, became essential reading and an indispensable reference book for army surgeons for 50 years. By the time of the Crimean War (1853–6) most of his teaching on the treatment of battle injuries had been accepted as standard practice. 'It was the mouse against the mountain', he said, 'I had every surgeon in that army against me, except for those who served under me, and everyone throughout all Europe'.[1]

In 1855, one year before his death, he gave a lecture at the Royal College of Surgeons of England which described the advances in surgical treatment made during the Crimean War and these had been incorporated in a new 6th edition of the book, which had a larger and more rapid sale than any other work at that time. All medical officers in the army were instructed to purchase a copy at their own expense, as it was the only book of practical instruction available.[2] Furthermore, Guthrie presented one free copy to every regiment in the British army and to all the principal officers in the East India Company. Even in 1916 during World War I the book was still being consulted, and the librarian of the Medical Society of London said that the *Commentaries* had been repeatedly borrowed by army surgeons, such was its reputation.[3]

Ballingall's *Outline of Military Surgery*, published in 1852 and a product of the eminent Edinburgh School where a Chair of Military Surgery had been established, was perhaps considered a rival publication to the *Commentaries* but large sections of it were devoted to preventive military surgery rather than pure surgical technique. The purely surgical sections were largely based on Guthrie's work, to which due acknowledgement was given.

One of Guthrie's last labours of love in connection with military surgery was the preparation of the Crimean Reports which appeared in *The Lancet* and in which the doctrines of former years had been tested and tried by recent practice.[4]

Guthrie continuously kept abreast of the latest developments in all branches of surgery, including eye and bladder surgery (see Chapters 13 and 18) and he was one of the first London surgeons to use a stethoscope ('unremitting attention in the use of the stethoscope', he wrote in 1848 in *Wounds and Injuries of the Chest*.[5] From the 1850s onwards he welcomed the use of chloroform in amputations.

The last letter that Guthrie wrote was to the Minister of War and in it he requested that a soldier of the 63rd Regiment who had been wounded in the Crimean War and who was soon to be discharged from Chatham Hospital following an operation in which six inches of bone had been removed from his thigh, should find a home in Chelsea Hospital. This request was granted, though Guthrie did not live to know the decision.[6] This letter was typical of Guthrie's long-standing concern for military personnel.

Retrospective view of his army service in the Peninsula

In 1849, seven years before his death, Guthrie looked back on his Peninsular War years in one of his lectures at the Royal College of Surgeons of England, and he said in a somewhat flowery way that:

> *[If he could]* now receive pleasure or satisfaction from the past, it would be from the position in which the past had placed *[him]* with respect to the future. Personally, I no longer derive either from anything; but there is, never-theless, a sort of mournful satisfaction in looking back to those days of the war in Spain and Portugal which were as joyous as they were laborious; and to find that the efforts which were made by those officers who served under my direction, and on many occasions almost beyond their strength, have enabled me to bring forward those improve-ments which have lately received the fullest corroboration by the Parisian surgeons in their late disturbances.

He then went on to write that he had:

> Recommended nothing which was not tried, and as far as I may venture to think, perfected under my own eye. If I have failed on any occasion it has been through inadvertence, not by design, and I shall most willingly efface it.[7]

This is another example of his, perhaps surprising, humility.

If he had disagreed with any of his contemporaries he had been careful in his lectures to avoid causing any offence.

Why was Guthrie so successful?

Guthrie's elder sister had inherited £10 000 (£656 350 in 2006) on her marriage[8] but Guthrie had not been so fortunate as his father's fortune was later lost (see Chapter 1, p. 2) and he had to rely on his own efforts and obvious natural practical and administrative ability, which he had so ably demonstrated during the Peninsular War. In addition he was very ambitious. The army medical service had provided a window of opportunity for young doctors without private means (see 'patronage' in Chapter 4, p. 71) and Guthrie was fortunate to have had the support of John Rush, Inspector–General of army hospitals, following his fortuitous accident as a young boy in 1798. He must have impressed the Inspector, who promised to provide Guthrie with a medical education, provided he entered the army 'as soon as he was capable of holding an appointment'.[9] This was at a time when army recruitment for doctors was high and the pay reasonable. It was opportune for the young Guthrie to take advantage of this.

But there was one other important factor which Guthrie described in the Introductory Lecture in the *Commentaries*:

> I had no quality save one, not possessed in a greater degree, perhaps, by all my seniors – an aptitude for labour, leading to the belief that little was done whilst anything remained to be done. I was always in the midst of every kind of work and perfectly willing to do everybody's business as well as my own, when they were not willing to do it, I always looked upon it as my individual property. It was this which now enables me to address you so didactically, or, as some may say, dogmatically; but which inclination for work I earnestly recommend you to adopt, having little faith in that great qualification which all are desirous of being supposed to possess, but which so few do possess, and which is called *genius*.[10]

Did Guthrie and Larrey ever meet?

Guthrie and Larrey sometimes had contradictory views on the treatment of war wounds, as mentioned by Guthrie in *Wounds and Injuries of the Arteries* and in *Wounds and Injuries of the*

Abdomen, both of which quote some of Larrey's cases. But at other times Guthrie agreed with Larrey's treatment. It is known, and it is evident from their comments on their case reports, that they respected each other's views. They probably corresponded with each other for Guthrie spoke fluent French.

There is no definite confirmation that they ever met, either in Guthrie's many books or articles on war injuries nor in Dible's biography of Larrey, which includes extensive quotations translated from Larrey's *Memoires*.[11] Guthrie states that after the battle of Toulouse 'the English and French surgeons visited each other and discussed the case histories of the injured' but he does not specifically mention either Larrey or himself.[12] Mary McGrigor's biography of her husband's ancestor[13] states that James McGrigor, accompanied by Thomson (another Peninsular War surgeon), visited 'my friend' Larrey and other French surgeons in Paris during the English occupation of that city after the Toulouse battle, but does not mention whether he was also accompanied by his close friend Guthrie. Dible's biography of Larrey states that they did not meet in Brussels after Waterloo as Larrey had to return urgently to Louvain (near Brussels) for family reasons'.[11] Richardson, who has also written a biography of Larrey, says that they did not meet.[14]

In 1826, well after the conclusion of the Napoleonic Wars, Larrey was given three months' leave to visit the United Kingdom. This extensive tour included Portsmouth, Dublin, Edinburgh and finally London, where he was received 'with signs of sincere fraternity' by Astley Cooper. He visited several London hospitals, including Chelsea, where he was welcomed by Everard Home. Astley Cooper personally accompanied him on a tour of the Hunterian Museum. He also watched several operations and was impressed by the 'calm deliberation, confidence and mastery' of London surgeons. He noted that 'they do not hurry the work of the knife as do some well-known French surgeons'.[11] It would seem inconceivable that these two eminent military surgeons did not meet each other in London but there does not appear to be any written confirmation of such a meeting. Perhaps Guthrie was not in London at the time of this visit?

Dible, a pathologist himself, thought that Larrey's recognition of thrombophlebitis and pyaemia was ahead of his time and he wrote that Guthrie had observed these changes at post-mortem but had failed to interpret them correctly'.[11]

Guthrie's family

Guthrie had a daughter, who did not marry, and two sons. His elder son, Lowry, entered the Church and was a 'gentleman of great promise'.[15] He was married, had one child and died in 1848 in Cambridge aged only 33 from 'apoplexy'.[16]

His younger son, Charles, who did not marry, succeeded his father at both the Westminster Hospital and at the Westminster Ophthalmic Hospital, despite Guthrie's antipathy to nepotism! 'Charles was a good surgeon and as an operator would, if the fates had not been against him, have taken a high place. He died at the very prime of life'.[17] Charles was very sociable. He resigned from his hospital appointments because of ill health and died aged 42 from 'ascites due to a liver complaint' (recorded on his death certificate as 'diseased liver, ascites')[16] only three years after his father. Like many sons he had been a 'cause of much anxiety to his father, who on more than one occasion had to pay for cattle shot on the Thames marshes under the impression that they were big game. He might have done well'.[18] Furthermore, confirming this anxiety, Guthrie had written to his daughter Anne on 13th December 1855, the year before his death: 'My Dear Anne, In making my will this day I wish you clearly to understand that I rely on your promise not to divest yourself of any portion of the property which I leave you in favour of your brother C. G. Guthrie, as you might just as well throw it into the sea' (Figure 7.1). There was clearly a problem with Charles and one cannot help wondering whether the 'liver complaint' from which he died was alcoholic cirrhosis.

Guthrie's first wife died on 18th September 1846 aged 65 years from cholera after two days' illness.[16] On 26th January 1856 he married Julia Wilkinson at the parish church St Ann,

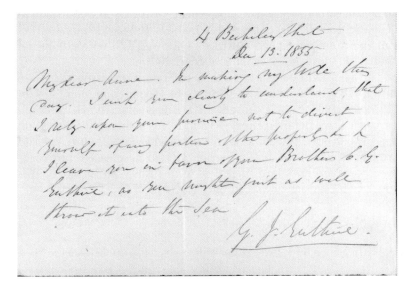

Figure 7.1 *Letter written to Anne Guthrie dated 13th December 1855. 'My Dear Anne, In making my will this day I wish you clearly to understand that I rely on your promise not to divest yourself of any portion of the property which I leave you in favour of your brother C. G. Guthrie, as you might just as well throw it into the sea'. (signed) G. J. Guthrie (RAMC 1759/5) (reproduced with permission from the Wellcome Library, London)*

Westminster.[19] She was aged 25 years, described as a spinster and was the daughter of John Wilkinson Esq, a term usually referring to a person of some status above a gentleman but with no formal title. *The Lancet* obituary notice stated that his second marriage was not generally known (presumably because of the age difference) and that he had a son between two and three years old;[20,21] this is corroborated by the 1861 census return (see addendum below).

The census for 1851 is interesting and shows that there were 12 persons ('those that abode in the house') residing at 4 Berkeley Street.[22] This included a housekeeper, a housemaid, two lady's maids, a nurse, a butler and a footman.

Name	Relation to head of family	Condition	Age	Occupation	Where born
George Guthrie	Head of family	Widower	65	Surgeon	London
Anne Leonora Guthrie	Daughter	Unmarried	39	None	London
Lady Bannerman	Daughter	Married	48	None	Halifax, N. America
Kate B. Guthrie	Daughter-in-law	Widow	29	None	Lincolns Inn
Mary Lucy Guthrie	Grand daughter	Child	3½	None	Cambridge

Lady Bannerman was born in Halifax, Nova Scotia (her age makes this to be 1803, the year before Guthrie's first marriage in Nova Scotia to a surgeon's widow). She is described as a daughter but she must have been Guthrie's widowed first wife's daughter by her previous marriage, i.e. a stepdaughter.

Guthrie had been saddened by the death of his wife in 1846 and in 1847 he wrote in the Preface to *Wounds and Injuries of the Abdomen* that he had suffered 'the greatest calamity which could possibly have befallen him'. To add to his sadness his eldest son died the following year at a young age. *The Lancet* obituary said that he 'might have had a baronetcy had he pleased' but these two bereavements had 'deprived him of any ambition of this kind' (which does not seem very logical).

Guthrie's death and will

Guthrie died suddenly from congestive heart failure at his residence, 4 Berkeley Street, Berkeley Square, London on 1st May
1856, his 71st birthday. For 20 years he had been 'affected with
a spasmodic cough which gradually increased particularly in
the winter and spring'.[23] During the previous three years he had
been increasingly dyspnoeic, so much so that he had been
unable to walk or shoot on his annual holiday in the country.
Latterly he had been carried up the stairs when attending the
College. The day before he died he had 'been dressed, received
friends and seen a patient. To the last, when not oppressed by
cough, his hand was as steady and his eye as bright as they had
ever been but of late years he had operated but little for fear of
being seized with a cough suddenly'.[23]

He left precise instructions for his funeral. He requested that
'nothing be paid to the newspapers announcing my decease
and that I may be buried in my niche at Kensal Green, being
carried there by a hearse and two led horses and followed by
one coach and two horses, without other additions, in particular
no feathers, walking undertakers, men on duty at the door'
(Figure 7.2). This was in striking contrast to his near contemporary Sir Astley Cooper, who had died in 1841, whose funeral
drew vast crowds and whose coffin was taken into Guy's Hospital
Chapel 'preceded by a plume of black feathers projecting
forwards from the coffin's head'.[24]

He was interred in Kensal Green Cemetery after, at his own
request, a private funeral attended only by his son and three
close friends: the Dean of Hereford, Lord Enniskillen and the
Hon. Mr Cole representing his old Peninsular friend Sir Lowry
Cole, to whom he was greatly attached. His daughter Anne did
not attend the funeral, as was the custom for women at that
time. His wife and elder son had predeceased him. Guthrie's
coffin resides in the catacomb beneath the main cemetery
chapel, adjacent to that of his wife and elder son Lowry. The
coffin is engraved with his name and date of death (Figure 7.3).
There is no memorial stone.[25]

His last will, dated 18th February 1856 and proved in
Canterbury on 14th July 1856 (Figure 7.4), bequeathed all his
estate, property and effects to his daughter Anne Leonora
Guthrie and appointed her as his sole executrix.[26]

After his death a marble bust of his head by B. Davis was
commissioned by his family and presented to the Royal College
of Surgeons (see Chapter 5, p. 76), which also owns an oil
painting of him by Henry Room (1802–50), presented by his
daughter in 1870 (front cover of book).[18]

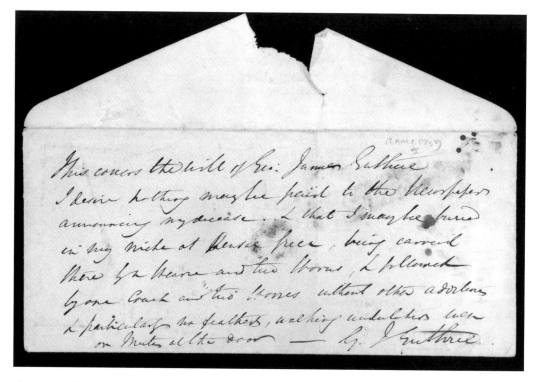

Figure 7.2 *Guthrie's instructions to be followed after his death. 'This covers the will of George James Guthrie. I desire nothing to be paid to the newspapers announcing my decease and that I may be buried in my niche at Kensal Green, being carried there by a hearse and two led horses and followed by one coach and two horses without other additions, in particular no feathers, walking undertakers, men on duty at the door' (signed) G. J. Guthrie. These instructions were written on an envelope (RAMC 1759/5) (reproduced with permission from the Wellcome Library, London)*

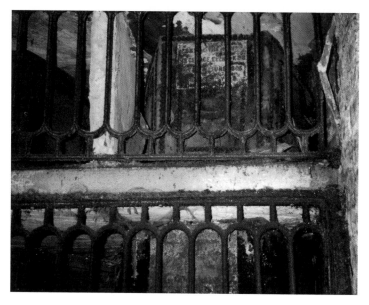

Figure 7.3 *Guthrie's coffin in the catacomb beneath the main chapel in Kensal Green Cemetery (Reference No. 6486, Catacomb B, Vault 124, Compartments 10, 11 and 12). The coffin is engraved with his name and date of death. There is, therefore, no memorial stone. (Author's photograph – a very difficult photograph to obtain as the niche is so high up)*

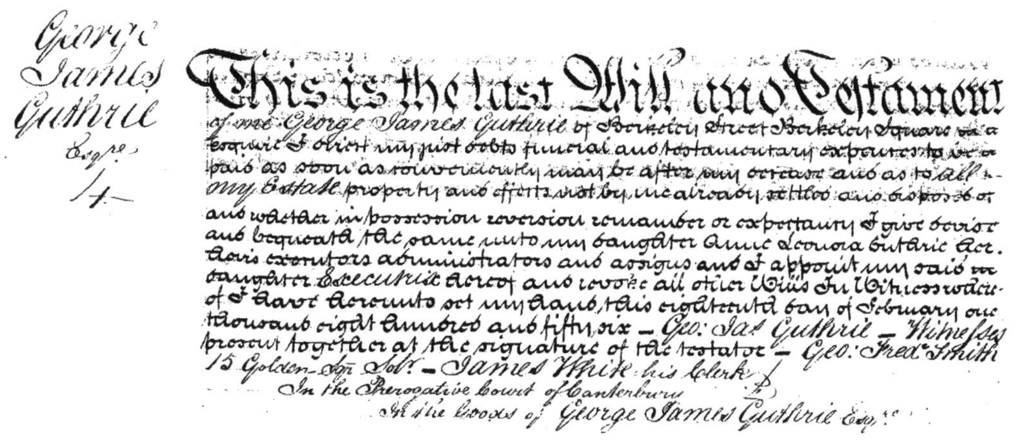

George James Guthrie Esqre. 1/4

This is the last Will and Testament of me George James Guthrie of Berkeley Street Berkeley Square in a ... esquire I direct my just debts funeral and testamentary expenses to be paid as soon as conveniently may be after my decease and as to all my Estate property and effects not by me already settled and disposed of and whether in possession reversion remainder or expectancy I give devise and bequeath the same unto my daughter Anne Leonora Guthrie her heirs executors administrators and assigns and I appoint my said daughter Executrix hereof and revoke all other Wills In Witness whereof I have hereunto set my hand this eighteenth day of February one thousand eight hundred and fifty six – Geo: Jas Guthrie – Witnesses present together at the signature of the testator – Geo: Fredk Smith 15 Golden Sqr Solr – James White his clerk

In the Prerogative Court of Canterbury

In the Goods of George James Guthrie Esqre

Figure 7.4 *Guthrie's will dated 18th February 1856. Public Record Office ref. 1172236*

Guthrie's wealth

Guthrie said in his Introductory Lecture in *Diseases and Injuries of the Arteries* that he had 'enjoyed a share beyond his deserts of private practice' and undoubtedly he had become very wealthy. This is always a fascinating subject, especially in the case of a member of a profession, but it is very difficult to assess Guthrie's real wealth. An in-depth Oxford University study of 19th century army surgeons' wealth and social mobility, published in 2006,[27] surprisingly gave the probate value of Guthrie's estate as only £450, but information from the online death duty register in the National Archives[28] states that the *duty* payable on Guthrie's estate was £22 273 – clearly these two figures are not compatible. Even if the estate's true probate value could be established, and even if it was low, such a lack of wealth on death would not necessarily indicate the size of Guthrie's assets or the quality of his lifestyle, for he had invested heavily in the education of his two sons, both of whom had been sent to Westminster School, following which one went to Cambridge to train as a clergyman and the other to Westminster Hospital to train as a surgeon.[29] He had settled £12 000 on his elder son on his marriage, £12 000 on his daughter 12 years before his death[27] and had also loaned £12 000 to the Duke of Buckingham, a loan which was never repaid (each of these three gifts amounts to over three quarters of a million pounds in present-day money).[30] Furthermore, other substantial gifts may have been made earlier to his three children.

It is interesting to note that Guthrie's contemporary Sir James McGrigor was said to be worth £25 000 when he died in 1855[31]

and Sir Astley Cooper an astounding half a million pounds (assessed in *The Times* obituary[24]).

Guthrie's legacy

George Guthrie revolutionized the treatment of war wounds in the early 19th century and the principles of his treatment became universally accepted and remained valid until the 20th century. He completely changed for the better the organization of the Royal College of Surgeons of England and gained for its members many of the privileges that they enjoy today. He was instrumental in the introduction of the important Anatomy Act of 1832. He became the historian of the Peninsular War through his personal recollections, described in *Compound Fractures of the Extremities* and in several other books on war injuries. Altogether, despite his several faults, he was a remarkable self-made man, appropriately and deservedly described as the 'English Larrey'.

Guthrie's memory was kept alive by the Guthrie Society at the Westminster Hospital which held an annual lecture in his name. Sadly the society no longer exists following the recent closure of the hospital. In this society every subject, save politics and religion, had been the subject of a lecture, demonstration or discussion. However, the army now awards a Guthrie medal to its outstanding civilian consultants – the first holder was Sir Stanford Cade, another Westminster surgeon, in the 1960s.

Guthrie's great great grandson

In the Guthrie archives at the Wellcome Library[32] there is an interesting letter from Lieutenant Colonel Ralph (Rollo) Gillespie dated 26th April 1972 to an unnamed general concerning the whereabouts of the papers and belongings of his two great grandfathers in the medical services. He wrote:

> My dear General, *[George Guthrie]* was a great great grand-father to my grandmother, who herself was the only child of an only son. He was killed when quite young by a falling tree. So all that exists came to me from both sides. It's not a lot now. My parents settled in Woolwich and their house was blitzed *[demolished by a bomb]* and they were killed. I was under orders for Normandy and had little time for the salvage. There was a good bit of looting I think, but some things in store.

There are portraits of Guthrie and a bronze relief portrait....
The Russians must have been impressed with his works
because I suppose around 1860 his daughter, when visiting
Russia (with my grandmother in tow), was presented with
a very fine brooch just because she was a relative....We
have a nice silver fruit dish presented to him in 1820 by a
grateful patient. He was a wealthy man and spent much of
it e.g. in founding the Westminster Eye Hospital.

In some of his letters from the Peninsula (now badly torn
and stained) he complained that pay and allowances were
six months in arrears and that the official rate of exchange
was scandalously low compared with the commercial
rate.

Rollo died in Australia on 21st February 1991 and his obituary
states that he had been private secretary to the Governor of New
South Wales for 10 years and that he left a wife and son.[33]

Addendum[34]

The 1861 census shows that Julia Guthrie, aged 30, was living at
Ringmere Green, Sussex, with her son George W., aged seven.

The 1871 census shows that Anne Guthrie was no longer
living in Berkeley Street and the 1891 census that she was now
aged 79 and living at Pool House, St Martin, Hereford with a
Mary Barnes, described as a widowed sister aged 84 and born in
St Johns, Nova Scotia. Is Mary Barnes the Lady Bannerman
recorded in the 1851 census, even though the name is different
and the ages do not tally between each census? Or is she Anne
Guthrie's stepsister-in-law? Also residing in the house were a
housekeeper, a lady's maid, a cook, a housemaid, a coachman, a
butler and a gardener.

Anne Guthrie died on 29th March 1893 aged 86 years from
bronchial catarrh.[35] Her will divided her estate between her niece
Lucy, wife of Colonel Williams Gillespie, and a friend Harriet
Nicholson.[35] No mention was made of Julia Guthrie's son, born
in 1854.

Notes and references

1. Guthrie GJ. *Commentaries on the Surgery of the War*, 5th edn.
   London: Renshaw, 1853, Lecture 1, p. 7.
2. Cantlie N. *A History of the Army Medical Department*. London:
   Churchill Livingstone, 1974, Vol. 2.

3. Grimsdale H. George James Guthrie FRS. *Br J Ophthalmol* 1919, **3**: 144–52.

4. Obituary. *Association Medical Journal* 1856; 389, 394 (precursor of *British Medical Journal*).

5. Guthrie GJ. *Wounds and Injuries of the Chest.* London: Renshaw, 1848, Case 69, p. 68.

6. *Lancet* 1856; **1**: 519–20.

7. *Lancet* 1849; **1**: 224.

8. Pettigrew TJ. *Biographical Memoirs of Physicians and Surgeons.* London: Whittaker, 1840, Vol. 4, p. 2.

9. Ackroyd M, Brockliss L, Moss M, Retford K, Stevenson J. *Advancing with the Army.* Oxford: Oxford University Press, 2006, p. 149.

10. Guthrie GJ. *Commentaries on the Surgery of the War*, 5th edn. London: Renshaw, 1853, p. 8.

11. Dible JH. *Napoleon's Surgeon.* London: Heinemann, 1970, pp. 242, 274–308. Also Chapters 28 and 29.

12. Op cit. ref 5, Preface.

13. McGrigor M (ed.). *The Scalpel and the Sword.* Edinburgh: Scottish Caledonian Press, 2000.

14. Personal communication, Richardson R.

15. Biographical sketch. *Lancet* 1850; **1**: 736.

16. General Register Office. Death certificates, refs. DYB 623655, 623844 and 623848. The York Probate Subregistry Office could not trace a will of Charles Guthrie, and it is likely that he died intestate.

17. Clarke JF. *Autobiographical Recollections of the Medical Profession.* London: Churchill, 1874, p. 261.

18. *Plarr's Lives of the Fellows.* Bristol: John Wright, 1930; **1**: 482–5.

19. General Register Office. Marriage certificate, ref. MXD 385963.

20. Obituary. *Lancet* 1856; **1**: 520.

21. No birth certificate for George W. Guthrie could be traced by Ancestors Genealogy Service. This may have been because the birth was not registered, as frequently occurred in the 1850s. Registration for *all* births was not made compulsory until about 1880.

22. Census return. Ref. HO 107/1476.

23. Obituary. *Lancet* 1856; **1**: 519–20, 556.

24. Burch D. *Digging Up the Dead*. London: Chatto and Windus, 2007, p. 12, 251.

25. Letter from General Cemetery Company, Kensal Green dated 23rd April 2001 – 'Margaret Guthrie buried 1846, the Reverend Lowrie Guthrie buried 1848'.

26. Public Record Office. Ref. 1172236.

27. Op. cit. ref. 9, p. 267.

28. National Archives. Ref. IR 26/2064.

29. Op. cit. ref. 9, p. 271.

30. Google – £10 in 1840 is worth £656 in 2006.

31. Op. cit. ref. 9, p. 292.

32. RAMC Archive 952, Wellcome Library.

33. South Wales Borderers Museum, The Barracks, Brecon, LD3 7EB.

34. Census returns refs. RG9/585 and RG12/ 2063.

35. General Register Office. Death certificate ref. DYB 678056.

[All the census returns, birth, marriage and death certificates will be given to the Wellcome library for storage with the Guthrie RAMC archive ref. RAMC 1759/5.]

CHAPTER 8

Contributions to surgery

I would remind you again how large and various was the experience of the battlefield, and how fertile the blood of warriors in making good surgeons.

(T. Clifford Allbutt, 1905)[1]

Much of the experience of older surgeons was gained in the service of Mars.

(G. Gordon-Taylor, 1952)[2]

War surgery

Guthrie revolutionized the treatment of war wounds following his extensive battle experience during the Peninsular War and at Waterloo.[3] This was against considerable opposition, even though it was known that Hunter's experience of these injuries had been very limited and John Bell's almost non-existent. But at that time the reputation of these two men, two of the leading surgeons of the previous century, was so great that an unknown surgeon's views had little impact, and it had been very difficult for Guthrie to refute their beliefs. In fact, as he so aptly said in 1853: 'it cost me the labour of seven campaigns and thirty years of teaching to overcome all those that were erroneous'.[4] Guthrie also wrote the same year:

At the commencement of the war in Portugal in 1808 there was little to depend upon but the opinions of Mr Hunter and Mr J. Bell. Mr Hunter had served for a few weeks in 1761 at the siege of Belle-Île *[off the coast of Brittany]* and it was much to be regretted that his opportunities were not sufficiently numerous to enable him to draw such inferences from them as would have left but little to desire. The greater part of what he did leave was not found to accord with the observations made by his successors; whilst the prestige attached to his name was so great as much to impede their progress on many essential points. Mr John Bell had not the same opportunity of seeing an enemy, even at a distance, as was enjoyed by Mr Hunter; and less reliance could be placed on many of the recommendations of a man of the greatest ability which was not supported by practical experience. They were found, therefore, on many points to be indefensible. The confidence placed in their opinions was nevertheless so great that it is only during the last year I have overcome all opposition, and that the principles and practice of the surgery of that war *[that]* I have published are admitted by all to be correct.[4]

Moreover, Hunter's observations had been based only on low-velocity musket and pistol ball injuries associated with little tissue destruction, and not on the more serious wounds from the heavier cannonballs which were used in the Peninsular campaign and, which Guthrie recognized, caused a different type of injury – 'there is an incalculable difference on many occasions between the effects of injury by cannon and of musket shot in the same part'.[5] Guthrie stressed that 'Hunter wrote from his knowledge of principles unbiased by a particular theory and from having [only] *some opportunities of practice*'.[5]

Concerning the controversial subject of primary (early) versus secondary (late) amputation, Guthrie accepted that the only way to confirm his opinion of the advantage of early operation, and its consequent lower mortality, would be to carry out what would now be called a clinical trial of the two procedures, but he said: 'I do not myself feel authorised to commit murder for the sake of experiment'[5] – a very rational decision.

In the first edition of *Gun Shot Wounds of the Extremities* (1815) Guthrie wrote in the Preface that he 'wished to preserve for the surgeons of the British army the credit for the improvements which they alone had introduced into the science and art of surgery'. But sadly he had to write in a later edition in 1827 that he had found that 'these improvements have not only been adopted, but pirated, and even by some advanced as something new by others, years after I had published them'.[6]

Guthrie's major contributions to war surgery are described below.

Straight splint to treat gunshot fractures of the arm and leg

These splints were advised in preference to the bent or curved splints which had been used previously and which had usually led to gross subsequent deformity. The position of a patient after a gunshot fracture of the thigh or leg was considered to be very important, both immediately after injury and during transport to base hospital – 'he should lie on his back and the limb should be straight,' Guthrie said. Guthrie ordered these straight splints to be sent out to Portugal from England in 1813.[7,8]

Ligation of both ends of an injured artery

The Hunterian policy of tying only the proximal end of an artery some distance from the wound allowed persistent back-bleeding to occur from its distal end due to collateral circulation, and this frequently led to a fatal outcome. Guthrie appreciated this complication at the battle of Albuhera after he had lost several men from secondary haemorrhage from this cause, and he realized that the haemorrhage could be prevented by an additional distal ligature. Until this time the opinion of Hunter had dominated surgical thought and the treatment of this type of haemorrhage had always been based on Hunter's proximal ligation only of an aneurysm.[9]

Primary amputation

Guthrie strongly advocated primary amputation for compound fractures and for joint injuries from missile wounds, before gangrene and probable later septicaemia occurred, as this so often led to greater loss of tissue and also of the more proximal joint, and, therefore, increased later disability. This was in direct opposition to Hunter's doctrine that amputation on the battle-field was more dangerous than amputation in hospital several days later. If amputation is not performed, Guthrie wrote, 'pain, redness and temperature of neighbouring parts constituting inflammation come on, which speedily runs into suppuration or gangrene, fever becomes more violent and frequently leads to death in the course of a few days'.[10] Furthermore, he wrote:

> The dangers attendant on secondary operation in military surgery are infinitely greater than those on primary operations; and the results of the practice of the whole of the surgeons of the British army, and of a great part of the French army, as given by Baron Larrey, ought to be decisive on this point and establish it as a law in surgery. That when amputation is indispensable it ought to be performed immediately after the injury, provided the state of the patient will admit of it; and it ought not to be delayed in any circumstances beyond twenty four hours with the view of obtaining a more favourable opportunity for its performance.[11]

He also emphasized that the 'pain of amputation is but trifling in comparison with the dreadful torture of a shattered limb, of suppuration, of ulceration, exfoliation and an unfortunate termination will more frequently occur than after amputation'.[11] A delay of a few hours was permissible only in cases of severe primary shock.

At the time of the Crimean War in 1855 he wrote: 'The advantageous results of primary amputation have been so firmly and fully established as to no longer admit of dispute'.[12]

Primary amputation had been advised by Wiseman and Ranby in the 17th and 18th centuries but this view had been superseded by Hunter's opinion. Guthrie was very logical in his reasoning and with his extensive battle experience he was critical of Hunter's opinion on amputation and wrote that he had 'examined the reasoning on which Mr Hunter's opinions were founded and I trust have proved it to be defective. That it was so ought to have been presumed when the facts were found to be opposed to the reasons'.[6] At the conclusion of the Peninsular War the teaching of Guthrie was accepted by Ballingall, Hennen, Thomson and other English surgeons for the rest of the 19th century.

Indications for amputation

Early in the Peninsular War all severely injured limbs were amputated immediately but Guthrie was very critical of these indiscriminate operations until a proper assessment of the viability of the limb had been made. Amputation 'was the opprobrium of surgery, as death was of the practice of physic,' he said.[13] He endeavoured to preserve a limb if at all possible, but if the indications for amputation were clear (severe damage to the limb or inadequate blood supply), he insisted it should be done within 24 hours, 'as soon as the first shock has subsided', and usually after a few hours. Injuries of the arm should be observed for 24 hours to see whether the arm was viable, as this would frequently avoid an unnecessary amputation (for an example see Chapter 2, p. 25). The whole question of amputation is further discussed in Chapter 10, pp. 164–5.

Excision of head of humerus or elbow joint rather than amputation

Severe damage to the head of the humerus or the elbow joint had usually been considered to be an indication for amputation of the whole arm. Guthrie did not agree with this policy, and in many cases he merely excised the damaged joint, allowing the arm, and in particular the hand, to be preserved. There would inevitably be limited use of the arm because of restricted joint movement in the shoulder or elbow, but nevertheless the limb would be valuable to the patient: 'leaving the limb for future use ... the importance of the arm is so great, and even a limited use of it so valuable, that much should be hazarded to save it, when there is a tolerably fair prospect of success'.[14] Such an operation could only be done by skilled surgeons who knew the position of the nerves and blood vessels adjacent to the joint to be excised,[15,16] and many army surgeons would not have had that necessary knowledge (see Chapter 19, Third and Sixth Lectures, and also Chapter 10, p. 166).

Erysipelas (streptococcal infection of the deep tissues)

Guthrie pioneered the treatment of this type of extensive and spreading infection by multiple skin incisions through the deep fascia to relieve the tension of the inflamed area (fasciotomy), which so often interfered with the circulation in the distal part of the limb (Figure 8.1). He introduced this operation after the battle of Salamanca and used it extensively during the rest of the Peninsular campaign.[17]

The above were Guthrie's major contributions to war surgery, to some of which there had been considerable opposition, and it was not until after the Crimean War (1853–6) and the American Civil War (1861–5) half a century later that they were all accepted as good practice. He was a pioneer of conservative surgery and, moreover, had little respect for established dogma unless it coincided with his own war experience.

Figure 8.1 *The operation of fasciotomy in the thigh (courtesy of M. Crumplin FRCS)*

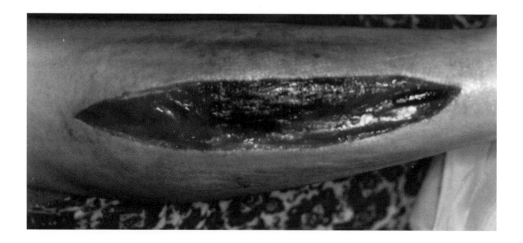

Guthrie's other contributions to war surgery are described below.

Exploration of the wound following severe arterial haemorrhage in a limb

This operation was first carried out after the battle of Waterloo when Guthrie ligated the peroneal artery rather than the more proximal popliteal artery – an operation which would have been likely to have led to distal gangrene and therefore an amputation. It is described in Chapter 4, p. 68. He also emphasized that an adequate collateral circulation was *not* necessarily present immediately after an acute arterial injury, as had been taught previously by Hunter; this was only true in the case of an aneurysm, which could therefore be successfully treated by proximal ligation.

Exploration of an injured artery

This should only be done if the artery *continued* to bleed.[18]

Penetrating wounds of the abdomen

Guthrie was one of the first to ban the use of purgatives following wounds of the abdomen, as this would, of course, increase peristalsis and encourage the onset of peritonitis. Previously, purgatives had always been part of an anti-phlogistic (anti-inflammatory) regime for this type of injury. Wisely, he also advocated the common-sense approach that food and drink should be restricted[19] (see Chapter 21).

Mineral acids

Nitric and sulphuric acids, together with vinegar, were used to destroy the necrotic tissue which occurred after the onset of what was called hospital disease – a collective term for gas gangrene, septicaemia and pyaemia.[20]

Statistical analyses of hospital admissions

Guthrie introduced statistical analyses to the army – they had previously been used in the navy. This was a natural development of his administrative work as Deputy Inspector–General of Hospitals after the battle of Talavera in 1809 and was used to support his views on the treatment of compound fractures and the related problems of what was called hospital disease[21] (see Chapter 2, p. 22).

Secondary amputation after onset of distal gangrene below the knee

The amputation should be performed just *distal* to the line of separation, the gangrenous tissue which remains being allowed to separate naturally. 'A joint will be saved and the patient has a much better chance of life,' Guthrie said.[22] Previously, an above-knee amputation had usually been advised for such an injury.

Compound fracture

Until the Peninsular War amputation had almost always been advised for a compound fracture at any site. Guthrie considered that every effort should be made to avoid amputation unless the bone had been very badly shattered. 'The object will frequently be obtained under good surgical treatment,' he said.[23] On the other hand, compound fractures of the thigh were much more serious and usually required amputation (see Chapter 11, Lecture 8, p. 178).

Use of a tourniquet

Guthrie was opposed to the use of a screw tourniquet (Figure 8.2) during an amputation – he thought it caused unnecessary tissue damage and pain, and, if not applied correctly, venous engorgement of the limb and therefore excessive bleeding. The artery could easily be compressed by an assistant. He had known the tourniquet to break on several occasions and rarely used this device after the battle of Salamanca in 1812.

Battle of Waterloo

After this battle Guthrie performed three operations which confirmed his leadership in British surgery and demonstrated his courage as a surgeon[24] – see Chapter 4, p. 66.

Venesection

Guthrie continued to advise venesection as part of the treatment of any major injury, as did many other surgeons until as late as 1896[25] (see Chapter 22, p. 267).

Guthrie emphasized three other aspects of war surgery in the sixth edition of the *Commentaries*, published during the Crimean War.

Figure 8.2 *A screw tourniquet – early 19th century (from Laffin J. Surgeons in the Field 1970. Reproduced with permission from the Wellcome Library, London)*

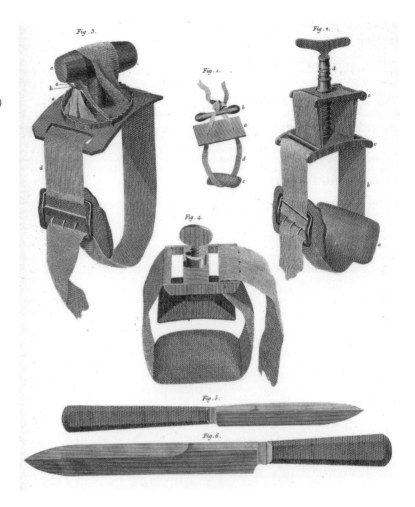

Finger examination of a wound

A penetrating wound should be examined with the finger to identify a missile, foreign material such as clothing, or bone fragments, so that they may be removed with forceps if possible. This was especially important if there was no exit wound.[26]

Closure of a wound

Contaminated wounds (as were most battle injuries) should not be closed immediately. He advised that 'the soft parts should be simply approximated by two or more sutures, the edges of the wound having a piece of lint or fine linen between them to allow drainage'.[27] This policy of incomplete wound closure is still the practice today.

Air embolism

The danger of air embolism in open wounds of the neck was noted, especially if the patient was upright – 'great care must be taken to prevent the ingress of air … as its admission in any quantity has occasioned sudden death'.[28]

Thoracic surgery

Guthrie must have had a special interest in chest surgery throughout his career for in 1848 he published *Wounds and Injuries of the Chest* (see Figure 22.1), the first book in the English language to be devoted entirely to this subject. This comprised 109 pages and included sections on auscultation and percussion, pneumonia, pleural effusion, empyema and emphysema. Indeed, for the 19th century, it was a truly comprehensive book on thoracic problems, both medical and surgical (see Chapter 22).

He and Baron Larrey made many contributions to the treatment of chest wounds, a subject which had hardly advanced since the time of Henri de Mondeville in the 14th century.[25] John Hunter had written very little on the chest, though he did advise drainage of a haemothorax.[25,29] Guthrie's contributions to chest surgery were first published in his *Commentaries,* and later as a series of articles in *The Lancet.*[30] They were based on his army and civilian experience, although he had written rather modestly in the *Commentaries* that he was 'fearful of approaching the subject'.[31] He thought that these injuries had always been treated badly in England and that many fatal cases reported to the coroner had 'died as much from maltreatment as from their injury. In some cases the unfortunate person had not a chance and died as much of his doctor as of his wound'.[31] As an examiner of the Royal College of Surgeons he found that many students did not know whether a chest wound should be left open or closed. He noted that French surgeons provided much better treatment for these injuries, and he wrote that 'there is, in truth, much to learn'.[31]

Six principles for the treatment of chest injuries were enumerated and each was very much ahead of its time. They showed a remarkable appreciation of basic physiology and also provided sound guidance for the management of these injuries with the facilities then available.

Immediate closure of an open wound

Previously chest wounds had often been left open but Guthrie appreciated the resulting danger of paradoxical respiration and consequent lack of oxygenation of the blood after these injuries. He therefore advised immediate closure by any means possible. He noted that *The Lancet* had reported a case in which the wound had been left open and the patient had died the next day, 'in all probability from its having been so done. The air had issued from the wound with each respiration with a whizzing noise and the patient had evidently developed severe paradoxical respiration'.[32] Guthrie did not claim originality for this policy for it had been advised by Valentin in the late 18th century, but it had been forgotten, as indeed it was again after the advice of Guthrie and of Larrey, until World War I.[25] Concerning chest closure he also said that 'the first object is to save life. After that, if time be given, the next will be to relieve the loaded cavity,'[33] i.e. treat a haemothorax or pneumothorax by removal of blood or air. This he did by reopening the wound or the insertion of a trocar and cannula a few days later, to prevent the lung being bound down by fibrin or what he called a false membrane.

Probing of a chest wound

This was almost a universal practice at this time and inevitably introduced infection. It was both unwise and unnecessary.

Conservative treatment

This was advised for many early cases of chest wound, unless very severe, an opinion still held during World War II.

Auscultation of the chest (discovered in 1819 after Waterloo)

This was considered to be vital in the diagnosis and management of haemothorax, and to decide when the blood should be evacuated – a far-sighted opinion for any surgeon, let alone a surgeon in the mid-19th century. Auscultation he described as 'unremitting attention in the use of the stethoscope'.[34]

Dependent drainage of an empyema

This was emphasized, though it should not be too low, as otherwise the abdomen might be entered, and this opinion he confirmed with descriptions of his abdominal dissections. He also emphasized the importance of early drainage to prevent rupture of the empyema into the lung, causing a bronchopleural fistula, which would delay healing. He considered it important to insert a rigid drain to prevent the drainage site closing too quickly, a fact not generally appreciated until 100 years later.[25]

Wounds of the diaphragm

These never unite but remain open, with the consequent risk of the late development of a diaphragmatic hernia. Guthrie was the first to point this out.[35]

Other branches of surgery

Urology

Lithotrity by a newly designed instrument introduced through the urethra was developed. Guthrie used this instrument for the first time on a soldier who had been transferred from Brussels to the York Hospital in London after the battle of Waterloo. A musket ball had been 'rolling about' in the bladder and had become encrusted and formed a stone. Previously these wounds had always been considered to be fatal due to later infection. The ball was removed from the bladder 'in the presence of a great crowd of persons', including James McGrigor and other military and medical staff officers. The operation was well described in *The Lancet*:

> The three-pronged instrument was introduced and the stone caught; it slipped and, on attempting to catch it again, the instrument was found to be wide open and immovable! Everyone was struck with horror. Mr Weiss *[the designer of the instrument]* sat down in a faint – he thought the instrument had been badly designed and that he had been accessory to killing a man. Captain Kater FRS, who was present with a great many others, held up his arms in great alarm. Mr Guthrie alone preserved that coolness, that presence of mind for which he has always been remarkable. He had previously considered and calculated upon all the difficulties he might encounter, of which this was one. Something was in the joint or sheath and how to disentangle it? Mr Guthrie forced the instrument open to its utmost extent thereby relieving it from a fold of the neck of the bladder which it had caught when it closed and was withdrawn. The patient, who saw the alarm of everybody at the occurrence, said 'You may cut out the stone, Sir, whenever you please, but you shall never put that three-pronged thing into me again'. The operation by incision a fortnight later was successful and the Duke of York was pleased to grant the patient's discharge as an especial favour. He, however, a few days afterwards enlisted again for the sake of the bounty, the examining surgeon never thinking of looking at his peri-neum to see whether he had been cut for the stone.[36]

Guthrie did not approve of either the transperitoneal suprapubic or rectal approach to the bladder, and, if this transurethral operation failed and it was necessary to 'cut for stone', he developed an extraperitoneal route through the lateral anal wall to the lower surface of the bladder (see Chapter 18).

Guthrie noted that a stricture could occur anywhere along the urethra and that an enlarged prostate was not the only cause for urethral narrowing. Many early 19th century surgeons advised caustic chemicals for their treatment but, in 1843, Guthrie preferred to use graduated silver sounds (see Chapter 18). He also described the *constrictor urethrae muscle*, sometimes called 'Guthrie's muscle' on the upper surface of the prostate – 'the urethra is thus enclosed between two muscular rhomboids,' he wrote (see Chapter 18).

He was opposed to the use of mercury for the treatment of syphilitic stricture of the urethra because of its unfortunate side effects, and preferred the use of potassium iodide (see Chapter 16).

Eye surgery

Guthrie was one of the first to *remove* a cataract rather than to use the traditional technique of 'couching' (displacement of the lens to one side with a needle). He strongly advocated this new technique, which had been developed by European surgeons, the use of which was initially opposed by most other surgeons in England.[37] In 1823 he published a comprehensive book on eye surgery, 200 pages of which were devoted to cataract and its treatment by extraction. A further book devoted entirely to the treatment of cataract was published in 1834 and this included a very detailed description of the operation, the precise technique for which he thought had not previously been described in order to preserve some secrecy about the operation. He also pioneered an operation to produce an artificial pupil by dividing part of the iris or sclera (see Chapters 12, 13 and 17).

A formidable operation in 1835

Guthrie's operative dexterity, for which he was justifiably well known and admired, was described by Pettigrew, an eminent surgeon and historian, in his *Biographical Memoirs of Physicians and Surgeons*. A tumour of the face was removed – the 'malar, lachrymal, the palate and the inferior turbinate bones were excised, the body of the sphenoid bone was scraped' and the posterior part of the tumour had to be dissected off the internal carotid artery. 'A thin, sharp chisel was used, in preference to scissors' for part of the operation. 'The coolness and precision with which this was done drew from all the hospital surgeons and teachers of anatomy who were witness of the performance, expressions of their admiration of the dexterity of the operator'[38] – a remarkable operation in pre-anaesthetic days.

Additional observations and comments

Neurology

Guthrie[39] described what would now be called the Babinsky reflex – 'tickling the soles of the feet will sometimes cause retraction ... when the limbs are apparently motionless'. He also noted that a cerebral injury will cause a contralateral paralysis – 'the mischief which gives rise to the loss of motion usually occurs on the side of the brain opposite to that part of the body which is paralytic'. The sign of a fixed, dilated pupil after head injury was also emphasized.

The heart[40]

Guthrie advocated auscultation of the heart after chest injury and noted the disappearance of pericardial friction and the diminution of heart sounds if a pericardial effusion developed. He agreed with Larrey's policy of pericardial drainage if 'suffocation is imminent. The relief obtained by the escape of a little blood', he said, 'may be efficacious. ... It is a choice of difficulties, and death from haemorrhage is easier than death from suffocation'.

Evacuation and care of the wounded

During the Peninsular War the arrangements for the evacuation of the wounded from the field of battle were very primitive, restricted and far behind those provided for the French army – unlike the French army (Figure 8.3), the British army had no proper stretchers and the casualties were carried in a blanket slung between two poles or in unsprung bullock carts (Figure 8.4).

Before the onset of the Crimean War Guthrie requested the Army Department to build two-wheeled, sprung ambulance carts (Figure 8.5), similar to those used by Larrey in the French army[41,42] (see Figure 11.2). A later version, with four wheels and drawn by two horses, was designed for the British army and was able to carry 12 casualties – nine sitting, two on stretchers on the floor and one stretcher slung from the roof.

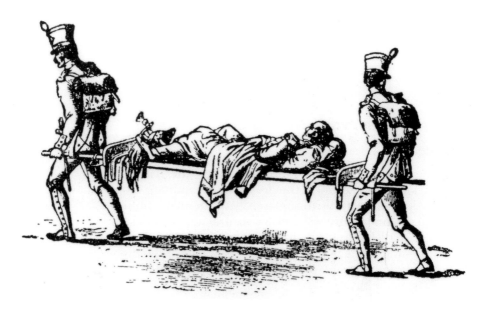

Figure 8.3 *Stretcher designed by Baron Percy, who had organized a regular corps of hospital attendants in the French army (from Laffin J.* Combat Surgeons *1999. Reproduced with permission from the Wellcome Library, London)*

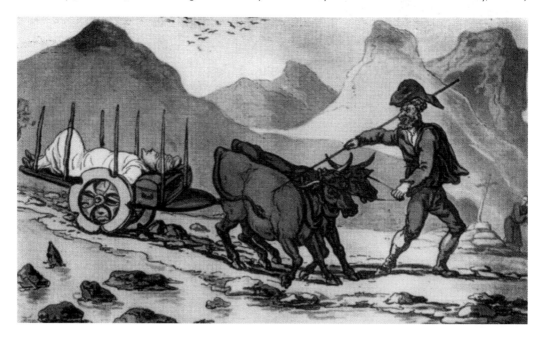

Figure 8.4 *Bullock cart (unsprung) used by the British army during the Peninsular War (from Howard M.* Wellington's Doctors *2002. Reproduced with permission from the Wellcome Library, London)*

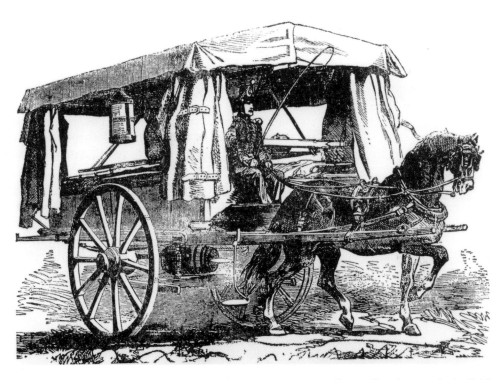

Figure 8.5 *Ambulance cart designed by Guthrie for use in the Crimean War (from Laffin J.* Surgeons in the Field *1970. Reproduced with permission from the Wellcome Library, London)*

The *Pamphlet on the Hospital Brigade*[43] was written shortly before the Crimean War and included Guthrie's 34 *Directions to Army Surgeons,* very briefly summarized below. It was required reading for all army surgeons and included very practical and clear advice – it concluded with a statement which emphasized the important advances in the treatment of battle casualties made during the Peninsular War and was typical of Guthrie's style of writing:

> The surgery of the British army should be at the height of the surgery of the metropolis; and the medical officers of that service should recollect that the elevation at which it has arrived has been principally due to the labours of their predecessors during the war in the Peninsula. It is expected that they will not only correct any errors into which their predecessors may have fallen but excel them by the additions their opportunities will permit them to make in the improvement of the great art and science of surgery.

The most important directions were:

1. The importance of water for injured soldiers.

2. Simple gunshot wounds only require the application of` a wet or oiled linen dressing, kept in place by sticking plaster.

3. Wounds made by swords or sabres should be 'treated principally by position' and ligatures inserted through the skin only; e.g. a wound of the upper arm requires the arm to be kept at a right angle to the body.

4. If the chest cavity has been opened by a sword the wound should be closed by the skin only and the patient placed on the wounded side so that the lung adheres to the wounded area.

5. Haemorrhage from a chest wound may be from an intercostal artery or from within the chest (which he described as a 'surgical bugbear'). The artery should be exposed by an incision and the artery ligated or 'pinched by forceps until it ceases to bleed'.

6. The drainage of blood from within the chest should be encouraged but if the bleeding continues the external wound should be closed.

7. A gunshot wound of the chest should not be closed by suture but covered with soft oiled lint after removing 'extraneous substances. The ear of the surgeon and the stethoscope are invaluable aids; indeed, no injury of the chest can be scientifically treated without them'.

8. Incised and gunshot wounds of the abdomen should be treated 'in *nearly* a similar manner'.

9. In bladder wounds a catheter is usually necessary.

10. In gunshot wounds of the skull 'all extraneous substances should be removed'.

11. An arm should rarely be amputated, except after a cannon shot. The head of the humerus or the elbow joint should be excised, with preservation of the arm.

12. A hand should never be amputated unless most of it has been destroyed. A thumb and one finger should be preserved if at all possible.

13. The head of the femur should be excised if broken, and amputation of the hip only performed if the fracture extends some distance into the shaft, or if the limb has been destroyed by cannon shot.

14. The knee joint should be excised when irrevocably injured, but the leg not necessarily amputated.

15. A gunshot wound of the mid-thigh with gross splintering requires amputation.

16. A leg injured below the knee rarely requires amputation unless due to a cannon shot.

17. A wound of the principal artery of the thigh associated with a gunshot fracture requires immediate amputation, but '*in no other part* of the body should amputation be done in the first instance': the artery should be ligated proximal and distal to the injury 'and events awaited'.

18. Gangrene rarely occurs in the arm, but frequently in the leg.

19. If gangrene has occurred below the ankle, delay may be advisable. But if it again spreads, then immediate amputation is required.

20. A stone, secured by a handkerchief, will often suffice as a tourniquet.

21. Hospital gangrene (infection) should be considered to be contagious and infectious.

22. Chloroform should be administered for all amputations.

References

1. Allbutt TC. *The Historical Relations of Medicine and Surgery*. London: MacMillan, 1905.

2. Gordon-Taylor G. The thoracic injuries of war. *Br J Surg* (War Surgery Suppl) 1952; **3**: 381.

3. Biographical sketch. *Lancet* 1830; **1**: 729–34.

4. Guthrie GJ. Introductory lecture. In: *Commentaries on the Surgery of the War*, 5th edn. London: Renshaw, 1853, p. 5.

5. Guthrie GJ. *A Treatise on Gun Shot Wounds of the Extremities*, 2nd edn. London: Longman, 1820.

6. Cited by Pettigrew's *Biographical Memoirs of Physicians and Surgeons*. London: Whittaker, 1840, p. 13.

7. Op. cit. ref. 4, 6th edn, p. 149.

8. Op. cit. ref. 3, p. 730.

9. Guthrie GJ. *On the Diseases and Injuries of the Arteries*. Longman, Burgess and Hill, 1830, p. 228.

10. Op. cit. ref. 5, p. 228.

11. Op. cit. ref. 5, p. 293.

12. Op. cit. ref. 4, 6th edn, pp. 59–60.

13. Op. cit. ref. 4, 5th edn, Lecture 5, p. 69.

14. Op. cit. ref. 5, p. 410.

15. Op. cit. ref. 5, p. 509.

16. Guthrie GJ. *Compound Fractures of the Extremities*. London: Churchill, 1838, p. 18.

17. Op. cit. ref. 3, p. 732.

18. Op. cit. ref. 4, 5th edn, p. 240.

19. Op. cit. ref. 12, 6th edn, p. 613.

20. Op. cit. ref. 4, Lecture 9.

21. Op. cit. ref. 5, p. 150.

22. Op. cit. ref. 4, 5th edn, Aphorism 29, p. 45.

23. Op. cit. ref. 12, p. 145.

24. Op. cit. ref. 3, p. 733.

25. Hurt R. *History of Cardiothoracic Surgery from Early Times*. London: Parthenon, 1996, pp. 107–9 and chapter 9.

26. Op. cit. ref. 4, 6th edn, p. 146.

27. Op. cit. ref. 26, p 138.

28. Op. cit. ref. 26, p. 291.

29. Gask G. *Essays in the History of Medicine*. London: Butterworth, 1950, pp. 145–54.

30. Guthrie GJ. Some of the more important points in surgery. *Lancet* 1853; **1:** 217–19, 239–40, 261–4, 285–8, 309–12, 331–4, 355–9, 377–9, 399–401.

31. Op. cit. ref. 4, Introductory lecture, p. 11.

32. Anon. Case of a wound penetrating the cavity of the thorax. *Lancet* 1825; **8**: 94–5.

33. Guthrie GJ. *Wounds and Injuries of the Chest*. London: Renshaw, 1848, Case 69, p. 67.

34. Op. cit. ref. 33, Case 69, p. 68.

35. Op. cit. ref. 27, p. 377 and ref. 4, p. 13.

36. Op. cit. ref. 3, pp. 733–4.

37. Grimsdale H. George James Guthrie. *Br J Ophthalmol* 1919; **3**: 144–52.

38. Op. cit. ref. 6, p. 20.

39. Op. cit. ref. 4, 6th edn, pp. 322–4. Also 5th edn, p. 310.

40. Op. cit. ref. 4, 6th edn, pp. 510–14.

41. Laffin J. *Surgeons in the Field*. London: Dent, 1970, p. 128.

42. Cantlie N. *A History of the Army Medical Department*. London: Churchill Livingstone, 1974, Vol. 2, p. 10.

43. Guthrie GJ. Mr Guthrie's directions to army surgeons. *Lancet* 1854; **2**: 155–7.

CHAPTER 9

Obituaries of George Guthrie

Seven obituary notices of George Guthrie (Figure 9.1) are included and, like so many obituary notices (even in the present day), there are a number of inaccuracies. The notice in *The Lancet* is probably the most accurate as it must have been written or commissioned by Thomas Wakley, the editor, who was a personal friend of Guthrie. The other obituaries repeat to some extent what was written in *The Lancet,* though there is additional information in the Royal College of Surgeons' notice.

Most of the information in these biographies has been included in the text of Chapters 1–8.

The Lancet *(10th May 1856)*[1]

Last week we mentioned in a few sorrowful words the loss the public, the profession and a large circle of personal friends had sustained in the death of Mr Guthrie. The particulars of the greater portion of his distinguished career have already been published in the first volume of *The Lancet* for 1850, so that in rendering a passing tribute to his memory we may refer to the personal traits of his character, rather than to the events of his long professional life.

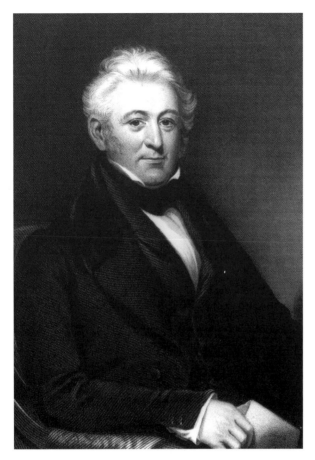

Figure 9.1 *Stipple drawing of George Guthrie FRS engraved by J. Cochran after a painting by H. Room, published by Whittaker and Co., Ave Maria Lane, in 1840 (in possession of the author)*

His early entrance into the profession; his precocious distinction as an army surgeon; his eminent services in the Peninsular War, of which he afterwards became the surgical historian; his success as a leading surgeon in this great metropolis for upwards of a quarter of a century; his triple presidency of the College which he joined as a boy of sixteen, are universally known to the medical public. Not so well known are the generous virtues and rare qualities of mind and heart which graced his private life, and the remembrance of which give at once poignancy and consolation to those who mourn him most deeply.

For the last twenty years Mr Guthrie had been affected with a spasmodic cough which gradually increased, particularly in the winter and spring. It was not, however, until the last two or three years that it troubled him much, but within this time he complained that it troubled him when going up more than one flight of stairs to see patients and felt troubled by not being able to walk and shoot as well as usual on his annual holiday. Otherwise he was strong and hale and he was often able to remark humorously that it was only his lungs which did not agree. Last autumn, instead of going away from London, he took a house in Willesden, where he went every afternoon, but this did not benefit him much, if at all. His cough and difficulty in breathing became worse during the winter months, still he was cheerful and free from pain, except during his paroxysms. He would have, during the twenty four hours and especially at night, several violent attacks of coughing, each of which left him faint for a time, but from these he would recover and in the intervals feel himself perfectly well. There was little or no expectoration, and the only distinct indications yielded by auscultation were those of a weak heart. Some pressure, as from an aneurysmal dilatation, was suspected but could not be positively made out. He saw patients during the winter and early part of the spring and attended the College, being generally carried up stairs. For a few weeks before his death he had rallied to some extent under the use of a freer quantity of stimuli than usual. Even the day before that on which his useful life terminated, he had been dressed, received his friends and had seen a patient. He had rested badly on the night of the 30th of April and on the morning of the 1st of May, which was his birthday, he expired in a faint following upon a fit of coughing. Death was not unwelcome to him. He had borne his last illness with Christian resignation; no one had heard a murmur from his lips and he waited patiently but expectantly for his release from trial. He had been attended throughout his illness by Dr Bright, Dr Elliotson, Dr Gairdner, Dr Hastings and Dr Hamilton Roe. His feeling had long been that he would not live over his birthday. To the last, when not oppressed by cough, his hand was as steady and his eye as bright as they had ever been, but of late years he had operated but little for fear of being seized with the cough suddenly.

In all that related to medical policy Mr Guthrie was staunchly liberal. He was for long the leader of the liberal party in the Council of the College of Surgeons, and the main author and promoter of almost every liberal measure which has marked the progress of the College in late years. At the same time he was devoted to the true interests of the College which he believed to be the greatest institution in this country. One of the last objects for which he strove in the Council was the institution of an examination in preliminary general education for students intending to pass the College. He had always contended for a reform of the obnoxious charter of 1843. He urged successfully with the Poor-law Board an increase in the qualifications and in the emoluments of Poor-law medical officers, and his heart was with the present Poor-law movement.

As an examiner he was supposed to be severe, and his brusque manner was little calculated to set a nervous student at his ease. He was certainly an object of some terror and apprehension to the grinding classes of students. He had, however, a most kindly feeling towards students, and he has been heard to declare, that when it came to depend upon his single vote, he never once in his life plucked a candidate. He attended his last meeting of the Court of Examiners on the 28th March.

In private life his manner was most genial and kindly, and to those who knew him best he was ever most gentle and attaching. As a friend he was most kind and constant, always thoughtful of the welfare of those whose interests he had at heart. His friends will ever have cause to remember him with affectionate gratitude. There was something of England, Ireland and Scotland in his blood, and certainly he possessed a rich vein of the wit and humour of the first, the shrewd keenness and penetration of the second, mixed and finely tempered with the cosmopolitan sympathies of the third.

As an author and thinker he was most industrious, and the vigorous and original powers of his mind will long impress the pathology and practice of surgery. In his meridian he was hardly more distinguished than as an anatomist. Forty years of peace could not dull the fire of the army surgeon. In 1855 he was as zealous as he was in 1815 for the sound administration of the army medical department. One of the last of his labours of love in connection with military surgery was the preparation of those Crimean reports which have appeared in *The Lancet* and in which the doctrines of former years are tested and tried by modern practice. His surgical works are well known but it is worthy of remark that his latest, the *'Commentaries'*, has had a larger and more rapid sale than any other modern work on surgery.

Mr Guthrie might have had a baronetcy had he pleased, but the premature death of his eldest son, the Rev. Lowry Guthrie, deprived him of any ambition of this kind. His professional income had for many years been large and he had accumulated a considerable fortune. Mr Guthrie was twice married, though the fact of his second marriage was not generally known. By his first marriage he leaves a daughter and a son, Mr A. Charles Gardner Guthrie. He also leaves a widow and a son between two and three years of age, who deplore his loss. Some misapprehension has been published about Mr Guthrie's extraction, which the following may correct.

Mr Guthrie was descended from an old Forfarshire family, the Guthries of Guthrie, one of whom married an Irish lady, and fought, and, it is believed, fell in the battle of the Boyne. His son farmed a small property he inherited near Wexford but, taking the wrong side of Irish politics, in one of the émeutes of the day, his house &c. were set on fire, and he and two of his sons were drowned by the upsetting of a small boat in which they were trying to escape from their pursuers. His eldest son had previously obtained a commission in the army but the rest were left destitute. The youngest, who was then of a tender age, found it difficult to gain a subsistence but, with the indomitable energy which afterwards so distinguished his son (the subject of this present article), he succeeded in earning for himself a respectable position. But he married unhappily as far as the temper of his wife was concerned and this drove him into habits of dissipation and excess. His son, who from the dissensions of his parents had an unhappy home, was early tempted to seek his own fortune, with what success the world knows. On his return from Spain he had the mortification of finding all his worst fears in regard to his father whom, with all his faults, he fondly loved, more than realised. He had fallen into the hands of a set of German quacks, who had dissipated his means and destroyed his character and health. He lingered only a year or two and his son had the happiness of witnessing his deep repentance and soothing his last sad but peaceful hours.

It may be a matter of satisfaction to Mr Guthrie's friends – and who had more and warmer? – to know that the last letter that he ever wrote was in accordance with his whole life. It was to the Minister-at-War, asking that a soldier of the 63rd Regiment, about to be discharged from Chatham and who had suffered and recovered from an operation in the Crimea never performed before (six inches of bone having been removed from the thigh joint), should find a home in Chelsea Hospital. His request was granted though he did not live to know it, but he expected it from the well known kindness of heart of Lord Panmure.

Mr Guthrie was buried at Kensal Green on Tuesday morning. The funeral was strictly private in accordance with his express wish that no parade should accompany his last obsequies. He had himself a peculiar dislike to attend funerals and he left express directions that no one should be invited to attend his own. He was followed to his grave only by his son Mr Charles Gardner Guthrie, The Dean of Hereford (who married one of his stepdaughters), Lord Enniskillen, and the Hon. Mr Cole, to whom he was greatly attached.

The Lancet *(17th May 1856): Marble bust of Mr Guthrie*[2]

The profession will be glad to learn that the eminent sculptor Mr Edward Davis, shortly after the decease of the late lamented Mr Guthrie, was sent for by the family of that distinguished surgeon and entrusted with the duty of taking a cast of his head and face and that Mr Davis is now engaged in modelling a bust for the family. It is to be hoped that the Council of the College of Surgeons, of which Mr Guthrie was thrice President, will not lose the opportunity of obtaining a good bust in marble of their late worthy colleague now that such excellent advantages are presented for having the lineaments of Mr Guthrie's features repro-duced with perfect exactness *[see Figure 5.1]*. We believe that no bust of Mr Guthrie yet made is entirely satisfactory but that very sanguine expectations are now expressed of completing one that shall be universally admitted as a good likeness of that truly estimable man and celebrated surgeon.

The Times *(2nd May 1856)*

The medical profession and the public generally will hear with regret that this distinguished surgeon expired suddenly of disease of the heart at his residence, Berkeley Street, Berkeley Square, yesterday morning, aged 71, having been born May 1, 1785.

Mr Guthrie was the only son of Mr Andrew Guthrie, at that time a celebrated chiropodist practicing in Lower James Street, Golden Square *[this is incorrect*[1]*]* with so much success as to give his only daughter a marriage portion of £10,000. Mr Guthrie commenced the study of the profession at the early age of 13 as articled student of Mr Phillips of Pall Mall, but he was specially placed under Dr Hooper, who afterwards became one of the ablest physi-cians and pathologists in London, and to whom Mr Guthrie was devotedly attached. In June 1800 Mr Rush, then Inspector–General, appointed the young student hospital assistant to the York Military Hospital, but Mr Keate, the Surgeon–General, objecting to these appointments being conferred on unqualified persons, directed the removal of all who had not been examined by the College of Surgeons. Before this tribunal therefore did young Guthrie present himself and on 5th February 1801 became a member of the College when not quite 16.

He was soon appointed an assistant surgeon to the 29th Regiment, commanded by Lieutenant–Colonel Byng, now Lord Strafford, who was only 22 years of age and Guthrie 16. Notwithstanding the youth of both it was always admitted that there was no regiment that was better commanded or better doctored. From 1802 to 1807 he served in North America; in 1808 he landed with his regiment on Mondego Bay, and on 17th August was at the battle of Roliça. The 9th and 29th Regiments furnished the greater part of the wounded, who for three days were almost entirely under Mr Guthrie's care. On the 21st of the same month he was at the battle of Vimiera. Mr Guthrie was present at the taking of Oporto and here he exhibited several examples of great presence of mind, especially in capturing a gun which the French artillerymen were endeavouring to drag through a lane, when the young doctor, being the only mounted officer present, made a dash at the gun and captured it; but what to do with it puzzled him; he therefore cut the traces of the headmost mule, a very fine one, brought her off as a trophy, and then sent a sergeant and a file of men to take charge of the gun until he could report its capture to Sir J. Sherbrooke, who was mightily amused at the doctor's capturing a gun by himself. He was present at the Battle of Talavera, at the retreat of the British army across the river Tagus – a most disastrous affair for the wounded, who were collected after several days' marching at the Convent of Deleytosa, near Truxillo, which Mr Guthrie called the slaughterhouse of the wounded of the British army from the loss of life which took place through the want of previous care and defective surgical knowledge. A want of space, however, prevents us following Mr Guthrie through all the Peninsular campaigns. It may be sufficient to state that on returning to London with a large amount of practical experience he commenced lecturing on surgery, which practice he continued for 30 years, receiving large attendances of the army, navy and the East India Company.

Mr Guthrie was elected assistant surgeon to the Westminster Hospital in 1823, and full surgeon in 1827. In 1824 he was elected a member of the Council of the Royal College of Surgeons at an earlier age than any other person so honoured – being only 38 years of age; and in 1833 was elected to the highest office, that of President – an honour again conferred on him in 1842 and 1855, being the only instance at present on record of a member of the Council holding this office three times. Mr Guthrie had also held the office of Professor of Anatomy and Surgery. For some time Mr Guthrie's health had been such as to occasion considerable alarm in the minds of his family and friends, arising evidently from a diseased state of the heart. A few days since he was considered much better and he contemplated sojourning for a short time in the south of France. On Wednesday evening he suffered much from a violent cough and on Thursday morning, at 5 o'clock, he ceased to exist. He leaves behind a son – Mr Gardner Guthrie, surgeon to the Westminster and Ophthalmic Hospitals, and an unmarried daughter.

Association Medical Journal *(precursor of the British Medical Journal) (10th May 1856)*[3]

This is a somewhat unsympathetic and critical notice following Guthrie's death.

The death of Mr Guthrie, which had long been anticipated by his medical friends, marks the close of an epoch, if we may so term it, in surgery. This gentleman was to his profession what his commander the Duke of Wellington was to the profession of arms – the able and vigorous defender of a system which has had its day. Mr Guthrie, though undoubtedly an able surgeon, was wedded to a style of practice which succeeded in the Peninsula but which, from a change in the nature of the human constitution, or from some other cause, does not succeed now; we allude to the practice of bleeding; sometimes to a heavy amount which he adopted even in cases when severe operations had been performed *[in fact, venesection continued to be practised by some surgeons even up to the end of the 19th century].*

With the decease of this able man we believe we have lost the last advocate of any note of a system which modern surgery, we think justly, condemns. The profession will regret the loss of Mr Guthrie for many reasons. He was of that old race of surgeons whose virtues we read of with approval in these more polite but not more true times. Honest, fearless and prompt, he was a good friend, or an opponent upon whom a man could rely – a virtue of no mean water in an age when the smoothest tongue often hides the deadliest venom. His work on Military Surgery is a monument to the clearness of his head and to the vigour and perseverance with which he pursued anything he undertook. Up to within a few months of his death he was engaged in writing it up to the last moment of the Crimean struggle; and of him it may be said, with Macbeth, that 'he died with harness on his back'.

In the same issue of this journal is an obituary notice identical to that in *The Times*.[4]

Proceedings of the Royal Society of London (1856–7)[5]

George James Guthrie was born in London on 1st May 1785 and died on the 71st anniversary of his birthday. He was descended from an old and respectable Forfarshire family, one of whom, his great grand-father, married an Irish lady and settled in her country. His father, a manufacturer of plaisterer and other surgical materials, raised himself from poverty to considerable wealth; but, late of life, was again impoverished, and left his son at an early age to seek and work his own way in the world. He was educated in boyhood by an emigrant French gentleman, M. Noel; and, when thirteen years old, he was apprenticed to the medical profession at the instance of Mr Rush, one of the army medical board. For a time he received his chief instruction from Dr Hooper, one of the most active pathologists of the day. In June 1800 Mr Rush appointed him a hospital assistant at York Hospital (a military hospital which then stood on part of the site of Eaton Square); and in the following winter he assisted Mr Carpue in teaching anatomy. In the beginning of 1801 he was to have been removed from his appointment with all the other hospital assistants who had not been examined at the College of Surgeons; and it gave proof of the success which he had already studied, and promise of the spirit which marked his later life, that he immediately offered himself for the examination. He passed and obtained his diploma at the College in February 1801; and in the next month, though not yet sixteen, was appointed assistant surgeon to the 29th Regiment with which, from 1802 to 1807, he served in North America.

In 1808, Mr Guthrie, having risen to the surgeoncy of his regiment, accompanied it to Spain; and from that time until the end of the Peninsular War (with the exception of a period of severe illness in 1810), was engaged in the most active service. He had a chief share in the charge of the wounded at the battles of Roliça and Vimiera; at the taking of Oporto; at Talavera and Albuhera; at the sieges of Olivenca and Badajoz; at Ciudad Rodrigo, Salamanca and Toulouse. In these fields of action he justly earned the highest reputation amongst the British military surgeons of his time; and all his writings prove that they were to him fields not only of action but of study.

In September 1814 Mr Guthrie was placed on half pay and commenced private practice in London. After the battle of Waterloo he spent a few weeks at the military hospitals in Brussels and Antwerp, studying chiefly those points of practice on which his Peninsular experience had left him uncertain. Returned to London, he commenced lecturing on surgery in 1816 and was appointed surgeon to the Westminster Ophthalmic Hospital, the establishment of which was mainly due to his exertions. In 1826 he was appointed assistant surgeon and in 1827 full surgeon to the Westminster Hospital. In the last named year he was elected a Fellow of the Royal Society. In the College of Surgeons he became a member of Council in 1824, President in 1833, 1842 and 1854, and during five years was Professor of Anatomy and Surgery [*Nearly all the foregoing statement is derived from an evidently authentic biography of Mr Guthrie in* The Lancet *of June 15, 1850].*

It would be very difficult to form a catalogue of Mr Guthrie's publications, for he was always active in publishing his knowledge and opinions on all questions which he had the opportunities of studying [*there followed a long list*].

Enterprise, activity and self-reliance were the chief characteristics of Mr Guthrie's mind. His intellect was acute and clear; his habits orderly and business-like; his constitution naturally robust, and till he reached old-age, capable of great exertion and endurance. These qualities, in circumstances so favourable to their exercise as those in the Peninsular War, quickly and justly placed him in the first rank of military surgeons, and accomplished a large amount of good in the medical department of the army. In after-life the same qualities, strengthened by success, ensured great influence for what he taught, gained for him a large private practice in surgery, and made him a man much to be considered in all the questions of professional interest in which he was engaged. His influence on the progress of medical science in his own time was that of an earnest advocate and an attractive teacher of whatever appeared simple and straightforward in practice, and of all surgical doctrines that professed to be based upon correct anatomy.

In the future history of surgery he will be remembered for his advocacy of the use of nitrate of silver in purulent ophthalmia, of large incisions in phlegmonous erysipelas, of acid escharotics in sloughing phagedaena, and for the skill and boldness of his treatment of gun-shot wounds. But, especially, his name will probably always be mentioned with honour for his maintenance of the general necessity of tying wounded arteries at the very seat of injury, above and below the opening. The usual practice had been to tie the artery at some convenient part above the wound, on the assumption that the arrest or diminished force of the circulation would allow firm closure of the wound, as it does the obliteration of an aneurismal sac. Few things in modern surgical works are equal in strength and clearness to the chapters in which Mr Guthrie proved the error of such an assumption and the advantages of his own mode of practice. In anatomy his best work was the bringing to general knowledge the musculi compressores urethrae, which, though described by Santorini, had nearly ceased to be recognised. In the medical department of the Army his influence for good was undoubtedly considerable. It may be difficult to enumerate the improvements that were made by him; but, as the last edition of his main work – the Commentaries on the Surgery of the War – will prove, he was to the very end of life urgent in promoting the efficiency of military hospital establishments, and in maintaining the reputation of the medical officers of the Army.

Plarr's Lives of Fellows of the Royal College of Surgeons *(1930)*[6]

Guthrie, George James (1785–1856). MRCS Feb. 5th 1801; FRCS Dec. 11th 1843, one of the original 800 Fellows; MD Aberdeen; FRS 1827.

Born in London on May 1st 1785. His grandfather, a Scotsman, served with the army at the Battle of the Boyne. His father succeeded his maternal uncle, a retired naval surgeon, as a manager for the business for the sale of lead plaster. Guthrie learnt French from the Abbé Noel when quite a boy and spoke it so perfectly that he was often mistaken in after-life as an émigré. At the age of 13 he accidentally came under the notice of John Rush, Inspector of Regimental Hospitals, who had him apprenticed to Dr Phillips, a surgeon in Pall Mall. He attended the Windmill

School of Medicine and was one of those into whose arms William Cruikshank – Dr Johnson's 'sweet-blooded man' – fell when he was delivering his last lecture on the brain on June 27th 1800.

From June 1800 to March 1801 Guthrie served as hospital mate at the York Hospital, Chelsea which then occupied what is now a part of Eaton Square. Surgeon General Thomas Keate issued an order that all hospital mates must be members of the newly formed College of Surgeons. Guthrie presented himself for examination on the day following the issue of the order, was examined by Keate himself and made so favourable an impression that he was at once posted to the 29th Regiment. He was then 16 years of age; his Colonel was 24 – but not withstanding it was generally agreed that no regiment was better commanded or better doctored.

Guthrie accompanied the 29th Regiment to North America as Assistant Surgeon, remained there until 1807, then returned to England with the regiment and was immediately ordered out to the Peninsula. There he served until 1814, seeing much service and earning the special commendation of the Duke of Wellington. He acted as Principal Medical Officer at the Battle of Albuhera though he was only 29 years old and one evening had on his hands 3,000 wounded with four wagons and such equipment as regimental surgeons carried in their panniers, and the nearest village seven miles away. He was appointed in 1812 to act as Deputy Inspector of Hospitals but the Medical Board in London refused to confirm the appointment on the ground of his youth. He was placed on half pay at the end of the campaign, began to practice privately in London and attended the lectures of Charles Bell and Benjamin Brodie at the Windmill Street School of Medicine. He hastened to Brussels directly after the Battle of Waterloo in June 1815, was received enthusiastically by his former comrades, amputated at the hip with success, extracted a bullet from the bladder and tied the peroneal artery by cutting down upon it through the calf muscles, the latter operation being later known as 'Guthrie's bloody operation'.

On his return to London he was placed in charge of two clinical wards at the York Hospital, with the promise that the most severe surgical cases should be sent to him. He discharged this duty for two years, during which he was amongst the first in England to use lithotrity. He also began a course of lectures which was continued gratuitously to all medical officers of the public services for the next twenty years. At the end of the first course, 1816–1817, the medical officers of the Army, Navy and the Ordnance presented him with a fine silver loving-cup appropriately inscribed. The cup has become an heirloom in the family of Henry Power, to whom it was presented by his last surviving child Miss Guthrie.

In 1816 Guthrie was instrumental in establishing an Infirmary for Diseases of the Eye, which became the Royal Westminster Ophthalmic Hospital, long situated in King William Street, Strand, next to the Charing Cross Hospital, but removed in 1928 to Broad Street, Bloomsbury. Guthrie was appointed surgeon and remained attached to the hospital until 1838 when he resigned in favour of his son C.W.G. Guthrie. In 1823 he was elected Assistant Surgeon to Westminster Hospital, becoming full surgeon in 1827, when the Governors made a fourth surgeon to mark their esteem for his surgical reputation and personal character. He resigned this office in 1843, again to make way for his son.

At the Royal College of Surgeons Guthrie was a Member of Council from 1824–1856, a Member of the Court of Examiners from 1828–1856, Chairman of the Midwifery Board in 1853, Hunterian Orator in 1830, Vice-President five times, and President in 1833, 1841 and 1854. He was Hunterian Professor of Anatomy, Physiology and Surgery from 1828–1932. He was elected F.R.S. in 1827.

He married twice and had two sons and one daughter, none of whom left issue. He died suddenly on his birthday – May Day 1856 – and was buried at Kensal Green.

Guthrie is described as a man of active and robust frame, keen and energetic in appearance, with remarkably piercing black eyes. Shrewd and quick, he was at times very outspoken and somewhat inconsiderate in regard to other people's feelings; but behind his military brusqueness was much kindness of heart. He was very popular as a lecturer, his lectures being full of anecdotes and illustrative cases, and his Hunterian Oration is memorable; it was given fluently and without notes, as was afterwards done by Sir James Paget, Savory, Henry Power, Butlin and Moynihan. He was noted for his coolness as an operator and for the delicacy of his manipulations. His unrivalled experience in military surgery, gained during the later years of the Peninsular War and at the most receptive period of his life, justly entitles him to be called 'the English Larrey'. It enabled him to advance the science and practice of surgery more than any other army surgeon since the days of

Richard Wiseman. Before his time it was usual to treat gunshot wounds of the thigh by placing the limb on its side. Guthrie introduced the straight splint. He differed from John Hunter in his treatment of gunshot injuries requiring amputation. Hunter was in favour of the secondary operation; Guthrie advocated immediate removal of the limb. After Albuhera he introduced the practice of tying both ends of a wounded artery at the seat of injury; Hunter contented himself with its ligature above the wound. Guthrie also advocated the destruction with mineral acids of the diseased tissues in cases of 'hospital gangrene'.

In connection with ophthalmic surgery he taught that the cataracting lens should be extracted, not 'couched', and he was one of the first to describe congenital opacity of the lens. He was heterodox in the treatment of syphilis for he recommended that mercury should not be used and his advice was largely followed by his pupils. At the College of Surgeons he was in favour of reform and did much to secure the passing of the Anatomy Act in 1832. He was opposed to the Charter of 1843.

A life-size half-portrait by Henry Room (1802–1850) hangs in the Secretary's Office at the Royal College of Surgeons *[reproduced on front cover]*. It was presented by his daughter, Miss Guthrie, in 1870. There is a bust by E. Davis, also presented by Miss Guthrie in 1870 *[see Figure 5.1]*; there are two copies of a fine mezzotint in the College Collection *[these could not be located in 2007]*. The plate was engraved by William Walker after Room, and was published by the London Publishing Co. on May 10th 1853. A crayon portrait by Count D'Orsay is in the Westminster Hospital *[this could not be located in 2007]*. There is also a clever but rather spiteful pencil sketch in the College Collection *[see Figure 5.5]*. It represents Guthrie lecturing on emphysema – May 6th, 1830 – 'Mr Guthrie's 11th Lecture' appears in the handwriting of William Clift below the sketch. It is initialled T.M.S. in the bottom right-hand corner. It was probably made by T. Madden Stone, Library Assistant in 1832, who was unfriendly to Guthrie – and not without reason.

A long list of publications follows.

Dictionary of National Biography *(1890)*[7]

Guthrie, George James (1785–1856), surgeon, descended from an old Forfarshire family, one of whose members settled in Wexford, was born in London on 1 May 1785. Having been early apprenticed to a surgeon, and served as an assistant in the York Hospital, Guthrie passed the examination for membership of the Royal College of Surgeons on 5 February 1801, when not yet sixteen. On March 1801 he was appointed by his friend Rush, then Inspector–General and member of the army medical board, assistant surgeon to the 29th regiment. After serving five years with his regiment in Canada he was ordered to the Peninsula where he remained (except for an interval in 1810) from 1808 till 1814, taking principal charge of the wounded at many important battles, and gaining the Duke of Wellington's special commendation. A graphic description of his Peninsular experiences, in which Guthrie often displayed the qualities of a soldier as well as a surgeon, is given in *The Lancet* for 1850, **1**, 726–36. After the battle of Salamanca he introduced the practice of making long incisions through the skin to relieve diffuse erysipelas.

In 1814 he retired on half pay and on returning to London diligently attended the surgical lectures of Bell and Brodie at the Windmill Street school, and Abernethy at St Bartholomew's. He found that his experience had enabled him to make considerable improvements in practical surgery. He had a further opportunity after Waterloo, when he successfully amputated a man's leg at the hip joint, divided the muscles of the calf to tie the main artery and extracted a ball from a man's bladder. Each of these operations was a novelty and the cases excited much interest

After the war the patients were sent to the York hospital, then situated where one end of Eaton Square now stands, and Guthrie gave lectures and took charge for two years of two wards in which illustrative cases were treated and exhibited. Here Guthrie was the first in England who used a lithotrite for crushing a stone in the bladder. At this time the Duke of York offered him a knighthood which he declined owing to want of means. Guthrie gave lectures on surgery from October 1816 for nearly thirty years which were open gratuitously to all the officers of the army, navy and East India Company. In December 1816 he founded an infirmary for diseases of the eye, afterwards the Royal Westminster Ophthalmic Hospital at Charing Cross, to which he was chief surgeon. An incautious remark in one of his lectures led to attacks on him in *The Lancet* (1850, **1**, 734) *[see Chapter 5, p. 76]*. Guthrie entered an action for libel which he afterwards withdrew, Mr Wakley, the proprietor of *The Lancet*, subsequently apologising and becoming Guthrie's firm friend.

He was elected assistant surgeon to the Westminster Hospital in 1823 and full surgeon in 1827; he resigned in 1843 to make way for his son Charles Guthrie as assistant surgeon. In 1824 he became a member of the Council of the Royal College of Surgeons, of which he was President in 1833, 1841 and 1854. He was Professor of Anatomy and Surgery from 1828 to 1831 and lectured on the principal subjects in which he had made improvements. As a councillor he succeeded in carrying numerous reforms in the College procedure and in its requirements from candidates for its diplomas; but he strongly opposed the charter of 1843. He died in London on 1 May 1856 and was buried in Kensal Green. He was twice married; by his first wife, Margaret Patterson, daughter of the Lieutenant–Governor of Prince Edward's Island, he had two sons and one daughter; the eldest son the Rev. Lowry Guthrie died before him; the younger, Charles Gardner Guthrie, became a capable surgeon but died in 1859 aged 42. He wrote *'Lectures on Ophthalmic Surgery'* and numerous papers on diseases of the eye (*Lancet*, 1859, **3**, 203) *[sic, but an incorrect reference]*.

Guthrie had an active and robust frame and keen, energetic features with remarkably piercing black eyes. He was shrewd, quick and sometimes inconsiderate in speech. His Hunterian Oration in 1830, delivered without notes, halt or mistake, was a notable success. His somewhat brusque somewhat military manner concealed much kind-heartedness and though dreaded as an examiner he never rejected a candidate by his unsupported vote. His lectures were very popular, being interspersed with many anecdotes and interesting cases. As an operator his coolness and delicacy of hand were of the highest order. His writings begin with 'Observations and Cases of Gunshot Wounds', published in the fourth volume of the *'New Medical and Physical Journal'* 1811, in which he insisted on tying both ends of a wounded artery. His celebrated work on gunshot wounds, published at the end of 1814, dealt especially with wounds of the limbs requiring amputation and advocated immediate amputation on the battlefield. The third edition in 1827 was enlarged and translated into German in 1821.

There follows a list of Guthrie's numerous publications.

Gentleman's Magazine *(June 1856)*

This obituary is almost identical to *The Times* obituary of 12 May 1856.

References

1. Obituary. *Lancet* 1856; **1**: 519–20.
2. The marble bust of Mr Guthrie. *Lancet* 1856; **1**: 556.
3. Obituary. *Association Medical Journal* 10 May 1856; 359.
4. Obituary. *Association Medical Journal* 10 May 1856; 389.
5. *Proceedings of the Royal Society of London* 1856–7; **8**: 272–4.
6. Plarr V. *Plarr's Lives of the Fellows*. Bristol: John Wright, 1930; **1**: 482–5.
7. Stephen L, Lee S. *Dictionary of National Biography*. London: Smith Elder, 1890; **23**: 375–6.

CHAPTER **10**

A Treatise on Gun Shot Wounds of the Extremities *(1815)*

A *Treatise on Gun Shot Wounds of the Extremities* was first published by Burgess and Hill in 1815, the year of the battle of Waterloo, and immediately after Guthrie had returned to civilian life. A considerably enlarged second edition was printed five years later in 1820 (Figure 10.1). It is a substantial book of 536 pages and includes five plates. It was the first of the many books to be written by Guthrie.

The following most effusive dedication of the book to 'Field Marshall His Royal Highness the Duke of York, Commander-in-Chief of all His Majesty's Forces', provides an insight into the quality of many of the members of the army medical service in the early 19th century. It also demonstrates the public attitude to royalty and the importance of patronage at this time.

> Sir,
> When your Royal Highness assumed the command of the British Army the higher situations in the Medical Department were filled by men from private life who had no further interest in it than what concerned their own immediate duties. The lower situations were held by men, who being nearly precluded from all hope of advancement, were frequently careless of improvement.
>
> Your Royal Highness soon perceived that little was to be expected from a body of men thus constituted; and by abolishing the sale of medical appointments, promoting from rank to rank according to merit, and by making the higher situations fair objects of ambition to all, imparted to them a vigour of thought and action to which they had hitherto been unaccustomed and brought the department to its present state of efficiency and public consideration.

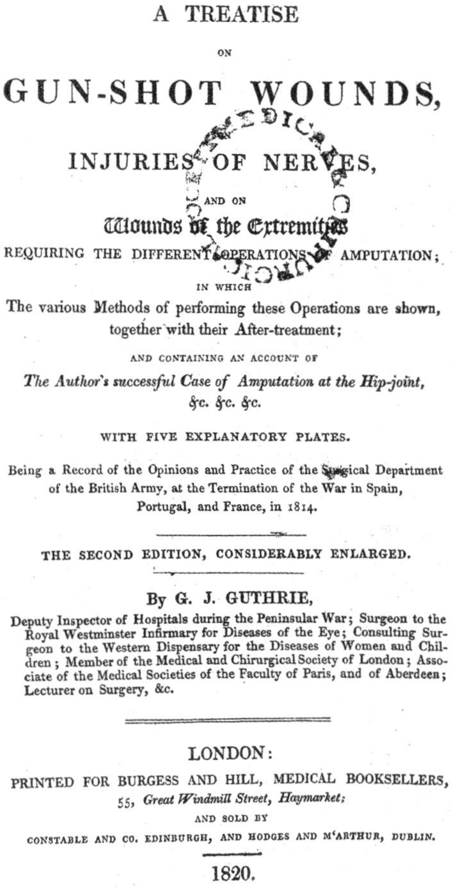

A TREATISE

ON

GUN-SHOT WOUNDS,

INJURIES OF NERVES,

AND ON

Wounds of the Extremities

REQUIRING THE DIFFERENT OPERATIONS OF AMPUTATION;

IN WHICH

The various Methods of performing these Operations are shown,
together with their After-treatment;

AND CONTAINING AN ACCOUNT OF

The Author's successful Case of Amputation at the Hip-joint,
&c. &c. &c.

WITH FIVE EXPLANATORY PLATES.

Being a Record of the Opinions and Practice of the Surgical Department
of the British Army, at the Termination of the War in Spain,
Portugal, and France, in 1814.

THE SECOND EDITION, CONSIDERABLY ENLARGED.

By G. J. GUTHRIE,

Deputy Inspector of Hospitals during the Peninsular War; Surgeon to the
Royal Westminster Infirmary for Diseases of the Eye; Consulting Surgeon to the Western Dispensary for the Diseases of Women and Children ; Member of the Medical and Chirurgical Society of London ; Associate of the Medical Societies of the Faculty of Paris, and of Aberdeen;
Lecturer on Surgery, &c.

LONDON:

PRINTED FOR BURGESS AND HILL, MEDICAL BOOKSELLERS,
55, *Great Windmill Street, Haymarket;*

AND SOLD BY

CONSTABLE AND CO. EDINBURGH, AND HODGES AND M'ARTHUR, DUBLIN.

1820.

Previous to this period the Medical Officers of the Army, strictly speaking, had done little towards the improvement of science. The many and important additions made to it since Your Royal Highness extended to them your gracious protection attest its power; and the benefits which the sick and wounded of the Army have received from their improvement and the amelioration of their situation, must be highly satisfactory to Your Royal Highness.

Military surgery, or that which more immediately relates to wounds and injuries inflicted on the field of battle has, during this period, undergone nearly a total change, and I thought it my duty to lay at the feet of Your Royal Highness the following work which records many of these changes and which is offered more as a humble tribute of that gratitude and affection for Your Royal Highness's person and authority, which is universally felt and acknowledged throughout the Army, than from any idea of the intrinsic merit which it may be supposed to possess,

By Your Royal Highness's devoted and very humble servant,

George James Guthrie

Figure 10.1 *Title page of* A Treatise on Gun Shot Wounds of the Extremities, *2nd edition published in 1820 (reproduced with permission from the Royal Society of Medicine, London)*

Part 1: Simple gunshot wounds

One hundred and fifty pages describe simple gunshot wounds, how much pain occurs and when – whether immediately after injury or later. Musket ball injuries may cause haemorrhage, contusion of soft tissue and bone fractures. There may be an entry and an exit wound or only an entry wound. If the latter, Guthrie noted that a musket ball did not necessarily travel in a straight line within the body but might ricochet and change direction according to the tissue it met, and this might make it difficult to locate the retained foreign body (Figure 10.2).

Guthrie also explained why his experience during the Peninsular War had shown that the treatment of soft-tissue

Figure 10.2 *Diagram to show how a musket ball may not travel in a straight line but may ricochet off adjacent tissue. It will travel from A to B, then to F, then to I and finally stop at L*

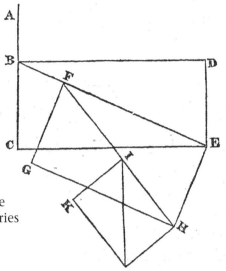

injuries which had been advocated by John Hunter and John Bell (Edinburgh) (in the third edition of *Discourses on Wounds* in 1812) and by Barons Larrey and Percy prior to the Peninsular War, was incorrect. These surgeons had not stressed the importance of incision of the deep fascia to prevent the later development of extensive infection. Guthrie related numerous case histories to confirm his opinion.

An axiom of military surgery is stressed:

> Whenever the constitution of a patient is implicated, whenever the powers of nature are considerably exhausted, the operation of amputation shall not be resorted to until the line of separation is fairly established.[1]

The 'old remark that gangrene often takes place without sufficient apparent reason, ceases in the same manner, and as readily recurs' is emphasized. His own experience confirmed that 'the prognosis should be very guarded until the mortified parts are completely separated'.[2]

The different types of gangrene and the effect of cold on the human body are discussed and Guthrie elaborates on this by comparing his own experience in Canada with that of Baron Larrey in Russia, whose opinion was quite often different from his own.

Guthrie instituted for the first time in the British army statistical returns of diseases, injuries and operations. These were to be of great value in the subsequent organization of medical services.

Part 2: Gunshot wounds accompanied by lesions of the larger nerves

A short section is devoted to case histories of patients with nerve injury and their management.

Part 3: Injuries of the extremities requiring amputation

Amputation of a limb is discussed at length and occupies 100 pages. Guthrie considered amputation to be the 'last resource in surgery by which an evil can be remedied that is incurable by other means',[3] but he agreed that there had been considerable disagreement on how soon after injury operation should be carried out. John Hunter, whose battle experience had been very limited, had stated in 1794 that 'nothing can be more improper than this practice' of primary (early) amputation,[4] and in his writings he had given several reasons for this statement.

Primary (early) amputation for severely injured limbs on the day of injury ('if the knife followed the shot')[5] had been advocated before the Peninsular War by Richard Wiseman (surgeon to King Charles II) in the 17th century, Ranby (surgeon to George II in the 1750s) in England and also by Le Dran and Larrey in France. On the other hand, John Hunter and most other French surgeons (Sabatier, Dessault and others) all advocated secondary (delayed) amputation. Baron Percy (France) had declined to give an opinion and maintained an equivocal attitude to the time of operation. These opposing views are extensively discussed. Charles Bell (John Bell's younger brother who 'considered that London was a good place to live in but not to die in'[6]) had published a book on wounds of the arm and leg in 1798 and was himself in favour of primary amputation, but his views were not generally accepted as it was well known that they were not based on personal experience, for he himself did not treat battle casualties until several years later at the battle of Waterloo. Guthrie was dogmatic in his opinion that immediate primary amputation was advisable except when the patient was in a state of shock, in which case 'a certain delay' was permissible.

Secondary (delayed) amputation was not advisable as it was so often followed by infection and its consequent high mortality. Numerous case histories are described to support Guthrie's own views and he concluded that:

> The dangers attendant on secondary operations in military surgery are infinitely greater than those on primary operations; and the result of the practice of the whole of the surgeons of the British army, and of a great part of the French army, as given by Baron Larrey, ought to be decisive on this point and establish it as a law in surgery.[7]

He then reiterated:

That when amputation is indispensable it ought to be performed immediately after the injury, provided the state of the patient will admit of it; and it ought not to be delayed under any circumstances beyond twenty four hours, with the view of obtaining a more favourable opportunity for its performance.[7]

Guthrie emphasized that 'the pain of amputation is but trifling in comparison with the dreadful torture of a shattered limb, of suppuration, of ulceration, exfoliation; and an unfortunate termination will more frequently occur in this state than after amputation'.[8] He also stressed that the bone should *not* be denuded of periosteum at the site of amputation as this would lead to bone necrosis, and he said that the saw should be maintained perpendicular to the shaft of the bone to prevent splintering.

A detailed description of the technique of amputation at the hip joint, of the thigh, foot and toes, is followed by a description of amputation at the shoulder, of the arm, forearm, wrist and fingers; this is well illustrated in five plates (Figures 10.3–10.5).

An operation which Guthrie had found to be of great benefit at the battle of Toulouse after cases of localized injury was excision of the head of the humerus or of the elbow joint. This was preferred to amputation as limited use of the forearm and hand was retained, a most valuable asset;[9] 'the importance of the arm is so great, and even a limited use of it so valuable, that much should be hazarded to save it when there is a tolerably fair prospect of success'.[10] This operation had first been advised by Boucher in France and White in Manchester in 1769 but it had been employed only very little in the British army, despite its use by Barons Larrey and Percy in the 1790s in Europe, and also by other surgeons in Canada and America in 1812–14.[11] Guthrie describes this operation which he again carried out at the York Hospital in London in 1815 – the subclavian artery was compressed against the first rib, and a flap of deltoid muscle was

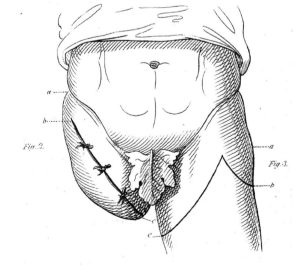

Figure 10.3 *Amputation at the hip joint.* Right, *line of incision.* Left, *appearance after operation*

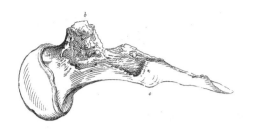

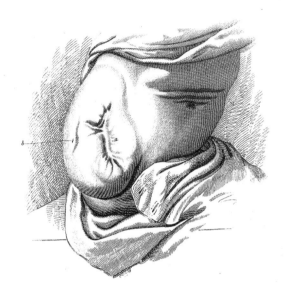

Figure 10.4 *Guthrie's first successful operation for amputation at the hip joint on François de Gay. The operation is fully described on page 332 of Guthrie's book (see also Chapter 4, p. 66).* Top, *the musket ball injury to upper end of femur.* Bottom, *appearance of the hip after the successful amputation*

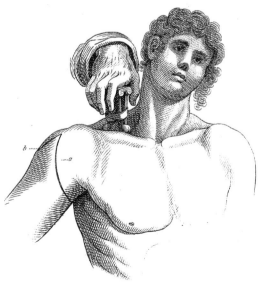

Figure 10.5 *Amputation of the arm – incision for amputation at the shoulder joint and site for compression of the subclavian artery by an assistant against the first rib from behind*

turned up to expose the shattered head of the humerus, which was then excised (Figure 10.6). The operation took three-quarters of an hour and six weeks later the soldier was discharged with 'little motion in the shoulder but with all the variety of motions of which the forearm and arm are capable'. Guthrie emphasized, however, that this operation 'should only be attempted by those who have a competent knowledge of the anatomy of the parts to be divided; whereas the more simple operation of amputation may be performed by anybody with little anatomical skill'.[12] At the battle of Waterloo Charles Bell had been very critical of this procedure.

The principles of this operation on the head of the humerus could also be applied to the elbow joint.

Two conclusions concerning amputation were emphasized:

1. No injury of the soft parts which is ever likely to occur authorises amputation as a primary operation, and 2. That when the bone is injured three different operations may be necessary – amputation, excision or the removal of splintered pieces of bone by incision.[13]

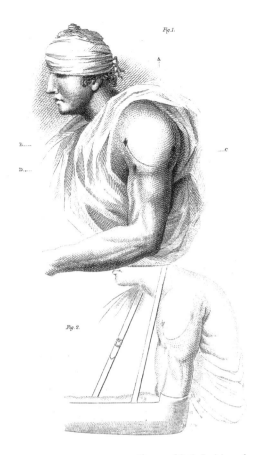

Figure 10.6 *Excision of head of humerus. Top, abscess surrounding shattered head of humerus, with anterior entry wound and posterior exit wound. Bottom, appearance after excision of head of humerus*

References

1. Guthrie G. *A Treatise on Gun-Shot Wounds of the Extremities.* London: Burgess and Hill, 1815, p. 116.
2. Ibid. p. 147.
3. Ibid. p. 191.
4. Ibid. p. 202.
5. Ibid. p. 226.
6. Guthrie D. *A History of Medicine.* London: Nelson, 1945, p. 269.
7. Op. cit. ref. 1, p. 293.
8. Op. cit. ref. 1, p. 295.
9. Op. cit. ref. 1, pp. 459–60.

10. Op. cit. ref. 1, p. 410.
11. Op. cit. ref. 1, p. 476.
12. Op. cit. ref. 1, p. 509.
13. Op. cit. ref. 1, p. 493.

CHAPTER 11

Commentaries on the Surgery of the War *(1815)*

Guthrie's most important book, *Commentaries on the Surgery of the War,* was first published in 1815 immediately after the battle of Waterloo. It reflected his experience of treating battle casualties during the Peninsular War. The book remained the standard English military text for half a century, was repeatedly updated as each new edition was published, and was said to have a larger and more rapid sale than any other work at that time. Furthermore, one free copy was presented to every regiment in the British army and to each of the principal officers in the East India Company.

Fifth edition

The fifth edition in 1853 (Figure 11.1) was dedicated to General Lord Viscount Hardinge, Commander-in-Chief of the Army, as was the custom of the times when patronage was so important (see Chapter 4, p. 71). It comprised 603 closely printed pages and 240 000 words – about three times the size of this biography – and followed the Hunterian tradition of being based on accurate observation of patients and the extensive use of Guthrie's own anatomical dissections and post-mortem studies. It covered all aspects of limb and blood vessel injuries, and head, chest and abdominal wounds, together with amputations, and it included 423 aphorisms concerning their treatment. Precise details of the treatment of each particular injury were included after each aphorism – these were followed by personal accounts of how, why and when Guthrie carried out this treatment, together with case histories which frequently described how the injury was sustained. They make fascinating reading. Perusal of these aphorisms shows that he also had remarkable insight into the management of penetrating head injuries, the signs and symptoms of brainstem compression (with an early description of the Babinsky reflex) and the physiological effects of haemothorax and of cardiac tamponade. The book included a comprehensive index (unusual for a mid-19th century surgical book) and a separate list of case histories of the various injuries. Most of the 31 lectures included many illustrative case histories and many were also published in *The Lancet* (1851–53).[1] Guthrie said that he intended the lectures 'to be almost aphorismal or expressed in the fewest possible words', though this is not exactly true when the text is read; like so much writing of this period it is somewhat verbose.

Sixth Edition

The last and sixth edition (published in England in 1855, the year before Guthrie's death, and in Philadelphia in 1862 during the Civil War in America [1861–5]), was larger, comprised 672 pages and included more illustrations. It also included the experience of other surgeons (Langenbech, Baudens, Luke and others – some now forgotten) gained in the Crimean War (1853–6) which was still in progress. Parts of the Preface are worthy of inclusion and show Guthrie's attitude to his great love of military surgery.

The demand for a 6th edition of this work enables me to say that the precepts inculcated in it have been fully borne out and confirmed by the practice of the surgeons of the army now in the Crimea in almost every particular. A fuller 'Addenda' shall be made from time to time as I receive further information

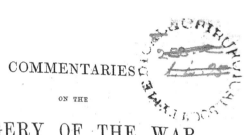

COMMENTARIES

ON THE

SURGERY OF THE WAR

IN PORTUGAL, SPAIN, FRANCE, AND
THE NETHERLANDS,

FROM THE BATTLE OF ROLIÇA, IN 1808, TO THAT OF
WATERLOO, IN 1815,

SHOWING

THE IMPROVEMENTS MADE DURING AND SINCE THAT PERIOD IN
THE GREAT ART AND SCIENCE OF SURGERY ON ALL
THE SUBJECTS TO WHICH THEY RELATE.

REVISED TO 1853.

BY G. J. GUTHRIE, F.R.S.

FIFTH EDITION.

LONDON:
HENRY RENSHAW, 356, STRAND.
1853.

Figure 11.1 *Title page of fifth edition in 1853 of* Commentaries on the Surgery of the War *(in the possession of the author)*

[an indication of Guthrie's continued involvement in military surgery right to the end of his life – this Preface was written the year before he died]. They have performed operations of the gravest importance at my suggestion, that had not been done before, with a judgement and ability beyond all praise; and they have modified others to the great advantage of those who may hereafter suffer from similar injuries. The precepts laid down are the result of the experience acquired in the war in the Peninsula, which altered, nay overturned, nearly all those which existed previously to that period – points as essential in the surgery of domestic as in military life. They have been the means of saving lives and of relieving, even if not of preventing, the miseries of thousands of our fellow creatures throughout the world.

I would willingly imitate the example of the best Parisean surgeons of detailing the improvements they have made … were it not that I might run the risk of being accused of gratifying some personal vanity, whilst only desirous of drawing attention of the public to the merits of the men who so ably served them in the last war, with scarcely a single acknowledgement of their services, except the humble tribute now offered by their companion and friend *[another example of his integrity and wish to acknowledge the contributions of others].*

4 Berkeley Street, Berkeley Square
October 7, 1855

New information in the sixth edition

Irrigation of the chest after gunshot wounds. Irrigation was 'often advocated and as frequently repudiated'. Guthrie considered that irrigation with water or diluted milk was beneficial and that 'pieces of cloth or bits of exfoliated bone often floated out'.[2]

Excision of head of femur. Six cases of the new operation of excision of the head of the femur, rather than amputation, are described – though only one survived.[3]

Amputation at the hip joint (the operation which Guthrie first carried out immediately after the battle of Waterloo in Brussels – see Chapter 4, p. 66) had been performed during the early part of the Crimean War with a 100% mortality, though in civilian practice there had been many survivors.[3]

Introductory lecture

The first part of this lecture is a diatribe against the poor administration of the army, a continual topic and complaint for the whole of Guthrie's life, and for the improvement of which he ceaselessly campaigned.

> The war minister ... should be the head of the doctors; the actual chief of the doctors should be his satellite, revolving round his centre of motion as if he were another Jupiter or Saturn. Then, and then only, will the calls of humanity be effectively complied with. A gentleman in civil life is no sooner appointed to an office, of whatsoever importance it may be and of the duties of which he knows perhaps but little, than he is presumed to be deserving of the confidence of the government and of the public, and it is granted to him. A clergyman or a lawyer is treated in a similar manner. No one disputes the integrity of an archbishop or of a chancellor but no one in a high official situation thinks of trusting a doctor. It is certainly not so acknowledged but it as certainly is the fact; and the medical department of the army will never afford to the public that quantum of good, of inestimable service it ought to give until this is altered; but when will a man be found at the head of the government strong enough in mind and warm enough with the feelings of humanity to do it?
>
> Inspector–Generals in the medical department of a certain age may always be placed in the same honourable list with Generals of Cavalry, all being full of science and learning but of little practical usefulness.

In addressing the junior officers of the medical department of the army Guthrie said in a way typical of his sometimes surprising modesty, but also of his constant desire for the truth:

> Follow implicitly the precepts I have laid down until you have reason, from your own observation or from that of others, to doubt. A little further experience will then enable you to confirm what I have said or to lay down in turn other principles which, whilst they supersede mine, may be of more service to mankind.

The remainder of the lecture is somewhat anecdotal but Guthrie does describe some general principles for the treatment of war injuries, in particular injuries to the shoulder or elbow. He compares the injury inflicted by a 16 oz English musket ball to a 20 oz French ball, and complains bitterly about the inadequacy of the unsprung wagons for the transport of British wounded compared to the sprung wagons used by the French and designed by Larrey (Figure 11.2).

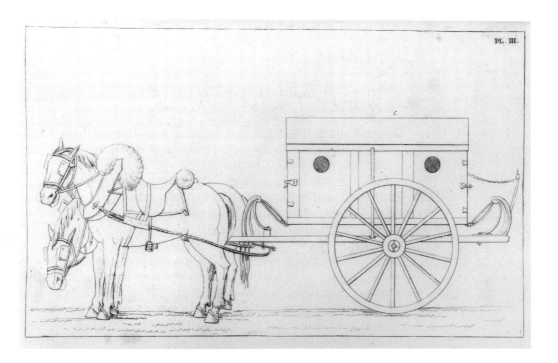

PL. III.

Lecture 2: Musket ball wounds

This lecture deals with the treatment of *musket ball injuries* in which the ball may traverse the body or be retained inside. The resulting damage to blood vessels and bones is discussed in general terms, as is the treatment of soft-tissue damage, the treatment of the subsequent infection two to three days later, and possible slough formation and its later separation. The application of leeches was considered to be more effective for deep than superficial inflammation. The difference between blunt (ball) and incised (bayonet) injuries is stressed.

Lecture 3: Erysipelas, gangrene, nerve injury and pain relief

The treatment of the dangerous condition of *erysipelas* (deep infection of the tissues) is discussed. The preferred treatment was by multiple long incisions down to or through the deep fascia (fasciotomy) to relieve the tension of the inflamed area – if this was not carried out, the casualty was likely to die.

Gangrene due to lower limb arterial injury, and when and at what level to advise amputation, is discussed. The distinction between dry and wet gangrene is explained. Injury to the axillary artery was considered to be less dangerous than injury to the

Figure 11.2 *A sprung flying ambulance (ambulances volantes) used by the French army (reproduced with permission from the Wellcome Library, London)*

femoral artery. Several case histories concerning *nerve injury* are included. *Pain relief* should be by the 'application of stimulants to the affected extremity, followed by narcotics'.

Lecture 4: Amputation, phlebitis and secondary haemorrhage

Amputation is discussed in general terms and is divided into primary (within the first 24 hours of injury) and secondary (several days or weeks after injury). If operation is delayed to the secondary stage it is frequently necessary to sacrifice the more proximal joint because of spread of infection to the soft tissues. After a lower leg injury this might require a more disabling above-knee amputation.

Inflammation of the veins (phlebitis) is divided into adhesive (or healthy, from which the patient usually recovers, and which would now be called thrombosis) or irritative (or unhealthy, which is usually fatal, and which would now be called deep venous thrombosis). The latter type may extend proximally within the vein as far as the lower inferior vena cava. Several detailed case histories are described, together with the post-mortem appearances in fatal cases, though pulmonary embolus was not recognized.

Secondary haemorrhage and its management are discussed. The lowest point at which external compression controls the bleeding is the preferred site for arterial ligation. If this fails amputation may be required.

Lecture 5: Amputation at the hip joint

> Amputation of a limb is the last resource and the opprobrium of surgery, as death is of the practice of physic [medicine], it being notwithstanding impossible to do impossibilities and save a limb or a life which can no longer be preserved. Art and science at that point cease to be useful.

At the beginning of the Peninsular War a great advance in amputation surgery occurred when it was realized that compression of the femoral artery against the pubic bone was possible. Until this time the loss of blood was 'so formidable as to be murderous'. Three assistants were required for the operation – one to compress the artery and two others to press on the outside of the skin flaps or the divided vessels. Since 1812 Guthrie had only rarely applied a tourniquet during this operation since 'it only did harm'. He condemned the practice of circular amputation and said that 'the parts so divided ought to be retracted as a whole to form a proper covering for the stump'.

He also condemned the former practice of 'nicking the periosteum and pushing it upwards' to leave space for the saw, as this so often led to necrosis of the denuded bone. He gave precise instructions as to how the assistants should hold the limb, the removal of which should be completed in two minutes, haemostasis being carried out more leisurely.

The major part of this lecture discusses *amputation at the hip joint*, first performed successfully by Guthrie on a French soldier in Brussels after the battle of Waterloo. Previous operations by Larrey and by Guthrie in Portugal had not been successful. Guthrie's technique is described in great detail (Figure 11.3), as also are the techniques of Brownrigg for hip amputation and of Luke's flap operation in the mid-thigh (Figure 11.4).

Lecture 6: Removal of the head of the femur and wounds of the knee and foot

Removal of the head of the femur may be required for scrofulous (tuberculous) disease or fracture through an external wound, though Guthrie himself had not carried out this operation. A preliminary study of the anatomy on a cadaver was necessary and the proposed operation is described in detail, the divided

Figure 11.3 *Amputation at the hip joint. Guthrie's operation. Right, (A) anterior superior iliac spine of ilium, (B) commencement of anterior incision continued to (C), the posterior incision joining the anterior one. Left, line of final suture (note that only three sutures are shown – Guthrie considered it to be important to allow for possible drainage of infected material after operation*

Figure 11.4 *Left, Brownrigg's hip amputation. Right, Luke's mid-thigh flap amputation*

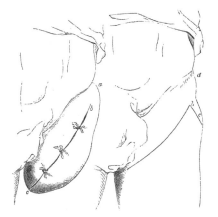

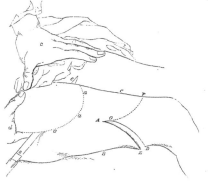

end of the femur being implanted into the acetabulum in the hope that its end would become rounded. Guthrie felt sure that this operation would be carried out at some time in the future. 'Surgery is never stationary and the surgeons of the present day must continue to show that it is as much a science as an art', he said.

Knee joint wounds inflicted by a musket ball and associated with a fracture require immediate amputation. Other injuries to the knee joint are discussed and only a few can be treated conservatively – the remainder also require amputation.

Amputation below the knee is described in some detail, either by the circular method or by a flap operation, in both cases leaving a stump about seven inches long (Figure 11.5).

Other operations described include excision of the ankle joint (Figure 11.6), the os calcis or the astragulus, as well as a more distal amputation of the foot anterior to the astragulus and os calcis, first described by Syme.

An operation by Wakley Jnr to remove the astragulus and os calcis only, with preservation of the distal foot, is described, leaving a less deformed foot than might be expected (Figure 11.7). The indication for this operation is not given but afterwards the patient was able to walk well with a high-heeled boot and to return to work. This operation under chloroform anaesthesia was reported in *The Lancet* on 1st July 1848. Removal of the astragulus only may be required (Figure 11.8).

Finally, a new type of artificial leg incorporating a 'rolling foot' is described (Figure 11.9), a great improvement on the wooden peg stump in general use up to that time.

Lecture 7: Amputation of the upper limb

Amputation of the arm is required much less frequently than of the leg. If the musket ball has damaged only the head of the humerus it is only necessary to excise the damaged bone (Figure 11.10), not the whole arm. The divided upper end of the humerus can then be implanted into the glenoid cavity of the scapula. Limited

Figure 11.5 *Below-knee amputation. Showing the line of incision A to F and A to E*

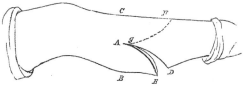

Figure 11.6 *Excision of the ankle joint*

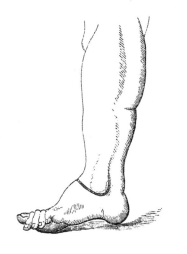

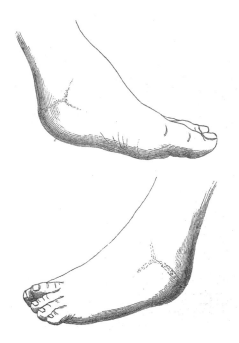

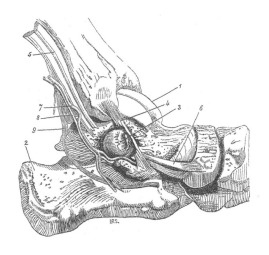

Figure 11.8 *Musket ball lodged in astragulus: (1) astragulus, (2) os calcis, (3) the ball, (4) torn ligament, (5 and 6) torn tendons, (7 and 8) posterior tibial artery and nerve (from the sixth edition of* Commentaries on the Surgery of the War*)*

Figure 11.7 *Excision of the os calcis and astragulus. Appearance after operation – the deformity is much less than might have been expected*

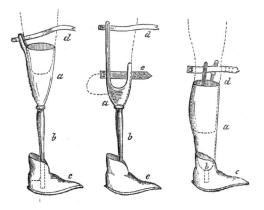

Figure 11.9 *Design for artificial limb after above- or below-knee amputation incorporating a 'rolling foot'*

movement of the arm, with preservation of the hand, will result – much to be preferred to amputation of the whole arm. This operation is described in more detail in *A Treatise on Gun Shot Wounds of the Extremities* (see Chapter 10, p. 165).

Amputation at the shoulder joint was perfected during the Peninsular War and was considered by Guthrie to be a very straightforward procedure, control of the brachial artery being by finger pressure until its actual ligation. The nerves were shortened to avoid their incorporation in scar tissue in the stump and consequent persisting pain. Depending on the extent of bone and soft-tissue damage the operation was completed with an internal and external flap or with one upper flap, each comprising skin and muscle. Detailed instructions for the procedure are given and Lisfranc's technique with a pointed double-edged knife is also described.

Amputation of the arm immediately distal to the humeral tuberosities is described and several case histories are included.

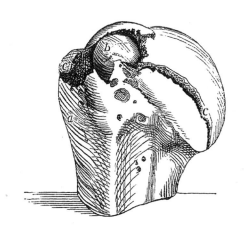

Figure 11.10 *Musket ball lodged in head of humerus. (a) head of humerus sawn off below the tuberosities, (b) the ball, (c) fractures of the head of humerus (from the sixth edition of* Commentaries on the Surgery of the War)

Other amputation techniques advised by Guthrie in the lower arm and at the elbow and wrist are described, as also are the techniques of Luke and Langenbeck.

Lecture 8: Secondary amputation and compound fractures

Secondary amputation is amputation one week or more after injury. In military surgery secondary amputation is usually required following infection of the wounded area, but it is not always successful due to frequent further infection and secondary haemorrhage. In secondary amputation the bone must be cut shorter and there will usually be excessive haemorrhage due to increased vascularity of the stump.

Compound fracture (i.e. associated with an open wound) is always the situation after a gunshot wound as it is inadvisable to close the wound as would be attempted after a civil injury. He advised initial conservative treatment for the arm but not for the leg. Of 12 secondary amputations of the leg carried out after the battle of Toulouse, only five survived. Of the 18 soldiers who recovered from their injury after this battle with preservation of their leg, 11 wished that their leg had been amputated and that they had a wooden leg.

At the battle of Toulouse the medical services had been good and the injured 'had every possible assistance and comfort from the second day after the action'. At this time there were 10 staff surgeons, 51 assistant surgeons and 'the whole worked from morning until evening with the greatest assiduity'. This was very different from the situation after earlier battles in the campaign when many injured lay on the field of battle for several days before any treatment became available.

Bone splinters are frequently associated with fractures due to gunshot wounds, and these splinters, unless removed, become infected, are associated with much new bone formation, and frequently form a sequestrum which must be removed. Many case histories are included, with an extensive discussion of their treatment, the preferred type of splint and how the injured should be transported. Luke's 'apparatus for compound fracture of the leg', in use at the London Hospital, is described in detail and is clearly the precursor of the Thomas splint used in the 20th century (Figure 11.11).

The lecture concludes with a *statistical analysis of hospital admissions* after the battle of Toulouse in 1813. The total of

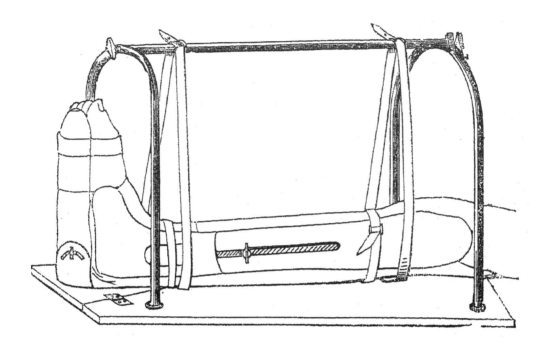

37 144 sick and wounded included in the returns for September to December 1813 was almost equal to the number of the whole British army. Guthrie considered that this demonstrated the 'labours of the surgeons of the army'. Statistical analyses were first used in the navy and were introduced into the army by Guthrie.

Figure 11.11 Luke's apparatus for compound fracture of the femur, as used at the Westminster Hospital. Note suspension for injured leg, splints and folding board to improve the patient's comfort (from the sixth edition of Commentaries on the Surgery of the War*)*

Lecture 9: Hospital gangrene

Hospital gangrene, 'the most destructive of diseases', was a collective term used to describe what would now be recognized as gas gangrene, septicaemia and pyaemia. In the early 19th century 'the peculiar nature of this poison' was not fully understood but it was appreciated that it was contagious and spread by 'the application of instruments'. Furthermore, it was also thought erroneously to be spread through the atmosphere. Mr Blackadder, a surgeon, accidentally infected himself whilst treating a patient; he recovered after two months and his dramatic personal description of this illness is revealing. 'Whilst examining the stump of a patient who had died from this disease I accidentally wounded one of my fingers with the point of a scalpel, but so slightly that not a drop of blood appeared.' Within 60 hours the wound became inflamed. Four days later he developed headache, nausea and frequent chills. A 'vesicle developed on a hard and elevated base; the surrounding integuments became tumified'.

The inflammation gradually subsided, the vesicle was opened, but it was two months before he completely recovered. (He was a lucky man – H. P. Nelson, a brilliant thoracic surgeon, died following a similar accident in 1936, despite multiple drainage operations and amputation of his arm.[4,5])

Tissue necrosis and sloughing were the characteristic clinical features of the disease and its natural history is described. At the battle of Salamanca Guthrie found mineral acids (nitric and sulphuric acid, together with vinegar) to be very effective for the removal of the necrotic tissue, a most important part of the treatment of this infection. The experience of several other surgeons is included. Sixteen recommendations to avoid and treat this infection included cleanliness, the avoidance of what would now be known as cross-infection and the use of mineral acids. The lecture concludes with a statistical analysis of cases of gangrene at Santander, Bilbao, Vittoria and Passages.

Lecture 10: The microscopical structure of arteries and of muscle

The six layers of the wall of an artery are described:

1. An *epithelial layer,* which changes with age, from 'strongly marked' cells in the young to the old, when 'all traces of cells and nuclei have disappeared';
2. A *fenestrated layer,* in which the fibres run in nearly parallel lines on a structureless membrane;
3. A *muscular layer,* the most important layer (the muscular coat of Hunter), which itself has an inner involuntary muscular coat and an outer elastic coat;
4. An *external coat,* also divided into an elastic inner layer and an inelastic outer layer.

The arteries themselves are nourished by *vasa vasorum* from neighbouring arteries.

The different type of collateral circulation after division of an injured artery and after an operation for an aneurysm is explained.

Lecture 11: Treatment of arterial injuries

Guthrie describes at great length why he disagreed with John Hunter's treatment of arterial injuries. Hunter's successful operation of ligation of the artery proximal to an aneurysm was not applicable to an injured artery, the treatment of which required proximal *and* distal ligation. This was entirely due to the lack of an aneurysmal sac after an acute arterial injury. This causation he suspected after the battles of Roliça, Vimiera, Oporto, Talavera and Albuhera but it was finally confirmed conclusively after the battle of Toulouse.

> This theory of Mr Hunter, then so new, so beautiful in itself, was eagerly embraced by all the civilised world; and surgeons were not content with applying it to cases of diseased or aneurysmal arteries but they extended it to cases of wounded arteries, to which the practice of the war in Spain proved it was inapplicable.

Guthrie emphasized that the collateral circulation associated with an aneurysm produced dark, venous coloured blood from the lower end of the divided artery and arterial coloured blood from the upper end. Guthrie concluded that:

> The presence of an aneurysmal sac in one case and its absence in the other is the essential difference destructive of the Hunterian theory for the treatment of aneurysm being applicable to wounded arteries.

The lecture continues with nine case histories of arterial injury and their treatment and then concludes with a discussion of the technique of arterial ligation and the structural changes which subsequently occur in the artery.

Lecture 12: Blunt and sharp arterial injuries

This lecture discusses extensively the treatment of blunt and sharp arterial injuries, in particular those of the femoral artery. This was amply demonstrated during the Peninsular War when, contrary to previous belief, it was realized that exploration of these wounds was feasible and that, if necessary, the femoral artery could be ligated without loss of the limb. Ligation of the more proximal external iliac artery did not arrest the haemorrhage. Numerous case histories demonstrated errors in the treatment of these cases. In some fatal cases the post-mortem examination showed that the haemorrhage usually ceased due to blood clot around the artery and not from contraction of the artery itself.

Guthrie also emphasized that it was important *not* to explore an artery unless it bleeds and, that if it is explored, the proximal *and* distal ends must be ligated to prevent back bleeding from the distal end.

Lecture 13: Gangrene due to arterial injury

The treatment of dry gangrene following blunt and sharp arterial injury is illustrated in many case histories, mainly involving the femoral artery but also the popliteal and subclavian arteries.

Lecture 14: Arterial injuries in the neck

Which artery is involved in arterial bleeding in the neck? It is always very difficult to identify the artery, whether it is the common, internal or external carotid artery, or even the vertebral artery. The complications which may follow ligation of each of these arteries are described and it is stressed that the common carotid artery must not be ligated. It is noted that Parisian surgeons were more advanced in the treatment of these injuries. As Velpau wrote: 'In haemorrhage from the neck, the mouth, the throat, the ear or the skull, everything should be done to reach the *branch* of the carotid which is wounded, rather than tie the carotid itself'. Numerous illustrative case histories, mainly civilian, are included.

Lecture 15: Arterial ligation for lower limb injuries

The precise technique of extraperitoneal ligation of the common iliac artery is described, an operation that Guthrie had successfully performed on two patients; the indication for the operation is not mentioned but it was probably for traumatic aneurysm. Techniques are also described for ligation of the internal and external iliac arteries (operations frequently performed in the early 19th century), and also of the more distal arteries. The techniques of Abernethy and Astley Cooper for ligation of the external iliac artery are described in detail.

Lecture 16: Ligation of carotid arteries and arteries of the arm

The precise technique for ligation of the internal and external carotid arteries is described, and also of the subclavian artery in the neck and the more distal arteries in the arm.

Lecture 17: Head injuries

Injuries of the head affecting the brain are difficult of distinction, doubtful in their character, treacherous in their course and for the most part fatal in their results.

A general discussion of head injuries is followed by their division into those from *concussion* and those from *irritation* of the brain.

The former are described by an expression used in our 'sister country' – 'that the life has been shook out of him' – and in these cases no apparent injury is visible on dissection of the brain at a post-mortem. The latter are characterized by headache and vomiting ('the stomach sympathises', he said).

Several case histories describe the later effects of a head injury, including that of haemorrhage into the substance of the brain.

Lecture 18: Further discussion of head injuries

Compression of the brain and its signs (eye signs, bradycardia, stertorous breathing and a positive Babinsky reflex) are all accurately described and illustrated by three case reports.

Middle meningeal artery damage, leading to an extradural haematoma and its treatment by trephination (burr hole) is described.

Fractured base of skull and contre-coup injuries are described in several case reports – they were not always fatal.

Lecture 19: Fractures of the skull

Fracture of the inner table is rare, although several case histories of such injuries are included and discussed.

Depressed fractures and their treatment are described. The question of the 'propriety' of converting a closed fracture of the skull into a compound one (by incising the scalp and elevating or removing the depressed fragments) is very important and controversial. Six such cases are discussed.

Lecture 20: Open and penetrating head injuries

Open and penetrating head injuries are discussed in general terms and many interesting case histories are included; in some cases there was a complete recovery.

Lectures 21–27: Chest injuries

These lectures all concern chest injuries and were incorporated in Guthrie's book on *Wounds and Injuries of the Chest,* published in 1848 (see Chapter 22), and the first book in the English language devoted entirely to this subject.

Lecture 28: Structure of the intestine and abdominal wounds

Following a description of the gross structure of the intestine and its three distinct layers – mucous, muscular and serous –

Guthrie describes the treatment of wounds of the abdominal wall, of those in which the injury has only exposed the internal viscera, and of those which have also caused visceral injury.

Guthrie condemned the former practice of the use of purgatives in the treatment of these cases. 'Absolute quietude' is essential with 'no food, minimal fluids by mouth and no purgatives'. He considered that penetrating wounds of the abdomen without injury to the viscera were not as dangerous as had been thought previously, provided that proper treatment was given.

Omentum, mesentery and intestine should all be replaced within the abdominal cavity after first cleaning them with warm water. The protruded abdominal contents should never be ligated and the peritoneal opening should never be enlarged.

Attempts to suture damaged intestine as early as the 15th century are described. For intestinal repair Guthrie advised a continuous all-layer suture, each suture separated by a 16th of an inch, with the edges of the intestine invaginated before drawing the suture moderately tight. He considered the outcome always doubtful, 'being dependant on many causes which the surgeon can neither foresee nor control'.

Many illustrative case histories are included.

Lecture 29: Further remarks concerning abdominal wounds

This lecture consists entirely of case histories of soldiers who had sustained penetrating abdominal wounds caused by bullets and swords. Surprisingly, most patients recovered. These case histories make fascinating reading and show the resilience of the human body, how well it can cope with injury and how well it can heal itself. In some cases bullets, 'portions of coat, flannel shirt and breeches' and musket balls, all of which had entered the abdomen, had later been passed *per anum*. In another case report an English officer had been shot in the abdomen but 'rode away with my bowel in my hand'. He recovered and later rejoined his regiment.

Lecture 30: Formation of artificial anus (colostomy) and wounds of the liver, stomach, spleen and kidney

Interesting illustrative case histories are discussed, many of which were bizarre, and many made remarkable recoveries from their wounds. These case histories also make fascinating reading.

Lecture 31: Wounds of the pelvis

Though frequently fatal, a soldier did sometimes surprisingly recover from these wounds, in some cases after several months. Many bladder injuries are described, not all of which proved to be fatal, though in many cases there was a temporary urinary fistula, the treatment for which was an in-dwelling urethral gum elastic catheter until the fistulous opening healed. Many other pelvic injuries are described.

References

1. Some of the more important points in surgery. *Lancet.* 1852; **1**: 87–9, 113–5 (Lecture 1 on types of injury), 165–8 (Lecture 2 on musket and cannonball injuries), 233–5 (Lecture 3 on erysipelas, arterial and nerve injuries), 417–21 (Lecture 4 on indications for amputation), 555–8 (Lecture 5 on techniques for amputation; issues 24 Jan–12 June); *Lancet* 1852; **2**: 47–51 (Lecture 6 on knee and ankle injuries), 117–21 (Lecture 7 on shoulder and elbow injuries), 187–90 (Lecture 8 on secondary amputation), 256–9 (Lecture 9 on hospital gangrene; issues 17 July–18 Sept).

2. Guthrie GJ. *Commentaries on the Surgery of the War*, 6th edn. London: Renshaw, 1855, p. 429.

3. Ibid. p. 645.

4. Hurt R. *History of Cardiothoracic Surgery*. London: Parthenon, 1996, p. 228.

5. Bucher T, Ellis H. Henry Philbrick Nelson MA, MD, FRCS (1902–36) – a promising career cut short. *J Med Biog* 2007; **15**: 127–30.

CHAPTER 12

Treatise on the Formation of an Artificial Pupil (*1819*)

This book of 209 pages (Figure 12.1) was published in 1819 because no other English work on eye surgery included 'the opinions of foreign authors in a connected manner'. Guthrie thought that the detailed discussion of these opinions made the book an important contribution to early 19th century surgical knowledge. In the Preface Guthrie wrote that he 'thought it right to combat the opinions of either the dead or the living with liberality. I have stated the facts on both sides as fairly as I was able and then drawn my inference from them'. The indications for the operation and its technique are described in detail and are extensively discussed (see Figures 13.4 and 13.5).

The whole of this book is included in a much more comprehensive book on eye surgery published in 1823 (see Chapter 13), which includes two plates showing the different types of artificial pupil and the instruments used by European surgeons for this operation.

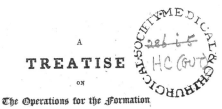

A

TREATISE

ON

The Operations for the Formation

OF AN

ARTIFICIAL PUPIL;

IN WHICH THE MORBID STATES OF THE EYE REQUIRING
THEM, ARE CONSIDERED;

AND

*The Mode of performing the Operation, adapted
to each peculiar Case, fully explained;*

WITH

AN ACCOUNT OF THE OPINIONS AND PRACTICE OF THE DIFFE-
RENT FOREIGN AND BRITISH AUTHORS WHO HAVE WRITTEN
ON THE SUBJECT.

With Two Copper-plates.

BY G. J. GUTHRIE,

Member of the Royal College of Surgeons; Deputy Inspector of Hospitals during
the Peninsular War; Surgeon to the Royal Westminster Infirmary for Diseases of
the Eye; Member of the Medical and Chirurgical Society of London; Associate of
the Medical Societies of the Faculty of Paris; Lecturer on Surgery, &c. &c. &c.

London:

PUBLISHED BY MESSRS. LONGMAN, HURST, REES, ORME, AND
BROWN; CALLOW, PRINCES STREET, SOHO; BURGESS AND
HILL, WINDMILL STREET; ANDERSON, SMITHFIELD; COX
AND CO. BORO'; HIGHLY, FLEET STREET; MESSRS UNDER-
WOOD, FLEET STREET: CONSTABLE AND CO. EDINBURGH:
AND HODGES AND M'ARTHUR, DUBLIN.

1819.

Figure 12.1 *Title page of* Treatise on the Formation of an Artificial Pupil, *published in 1819 (reproduced with permission from the Royal Society of Medicine, London)*

CHAPTER 13

Lectures on Operative Surgery of the Eye *(1823)*

This comprehensive and substantial book (Figure 13.1) was first published by Burgess and Hill in 1823, with a further edition in 1827. It comprised 517 pages and included five excellent plates (three in colour) which illustrate inversion and eversion of the eyelid and its treatment, the four types of cataract, the formation of an artificial pupil and instruments for eye surgery (Figures 13.2–13.6).

To summarize and describe this well-written book is impossible but it must have filled a gap in the surgical literature of the early 19th century; three more editions were published up to 1843. This book would fascinate anyone interested in the operative techniques of eye surgery in the early 19th century.

Preface

In the Preface Guthrie stresses that the eyeball itself is insensitive unless it becomes inflamed and he explains how the eyelid responds to a foreign body under its surface. He then goes on to say that prior to 1817 no lectures were given on diseases and surgery of

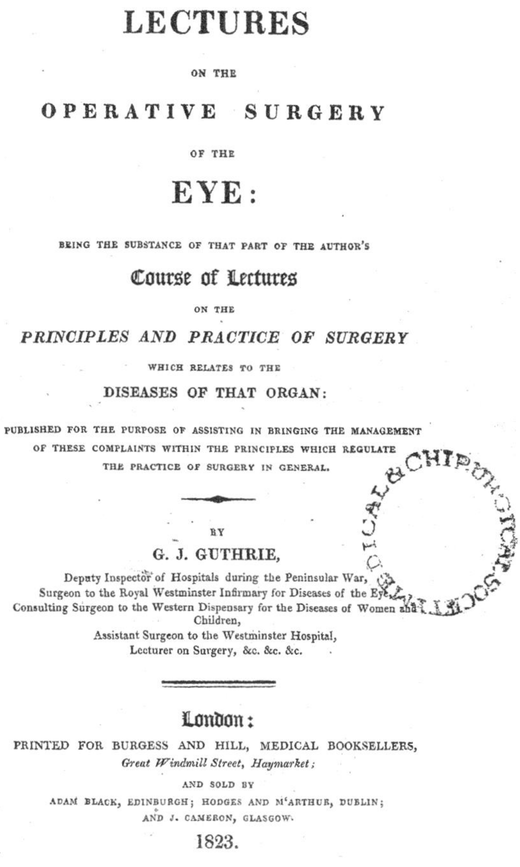

Figure 13.1 *Title page of* Lectures on Operative Surgery of the Eye, *published in 1823 (reproduced with permission from the Royal Society of Medicine, London)*

LECTURES

ON THE

OPERATIVE SURGERY

OF THE

EYE:

BEING THE SUBSTANCE OF THAT PART OF THE AUTHOR'S

Course of Lectures

ON THE

PRINCIPLES AND PRACTICE OF SURGERY

WHICH RELATES TO THE

DISEASES OF THAT ORGAN:

PUBLISHED FOR THE PURPOSE OF ASSISTING IN BRINGING THE MANAGEMENT OF THESE COMPLAINTS WITHIN THE PRINCIPLES WHICH REGULATE THE PRACTICE OF SURGERY IN GENERAL.

BY

G. J. GUTHRIE,

Deputy Inspector of Hospitals during the Peninsular War, Surgeon to the Royal Westminster Infirmary for Diseases of the Eye, Consulting Surgeon to the Western Dispensary for the Diseases of Women and Children, Assistant Surgeon to the Westminster Hospital, Lecturer on Surgery, &c. &c. &c.

London:

PRINTED FOR BURGESS AND HILL, MEDICAL BOOKSELLERS, *Great Windmill Street, Haymarket;*

AND SOLD BY

ADAM BLACK, EDINBURGH; HODGES AND M'ARTHUR, DUBLIN; AND J. CAMERON, GLASGOW.

1823.

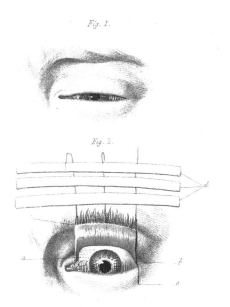

Figure 13.2 *Plate 1. Above, the cilia of both lids inverted, and below, an operation for inversion of the upper eyelid, showing (a) and (b) inner and outer incisions, (c) ligatures supporting eyelid against eyebrow, (d) strips of adhesive plaster fixing ligatures to forehead and (e) incision for inversion of lower lid (in colour)*

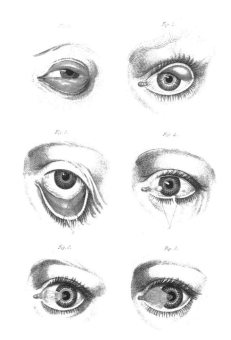

Figure 13.3 *Plate 2. Above, eversion of the lid before and after operation; middle, before and after operation; below, on left a membranous pterygium and on right a fleshy pterygium (in colour)*

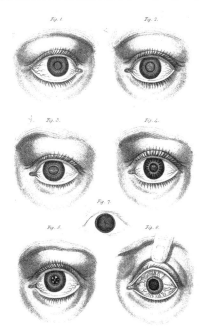

Figure 13.4 *Plate 3. Types of cataract and,* bottom right, *glaucoma (in colour) (detailed descriptions are included)*

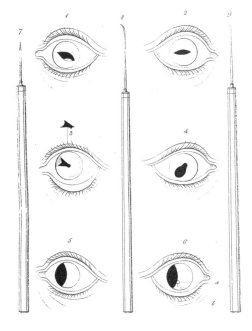

Figure 13.5 *Plate 4. The appearance of different types of artificial pupil, together with instruments for eye surgery (detailed descriptions are included)*

the eye as these were not considered to be part of a surgeon's training. Because of this attitude Guthrie and Dr Forbes, surgeon and physician, respectively, to the Royal Westminster Infirmary for Diseases of the Eye in Marylebone Street, Piccadilly, began a course of lectures soon after their appointment. Guthrie wrote that he:

> Avoided as much as possible entering into controversy; and where I have thought it right to combat the opinions of either the dead or the living, I have endeavoured to do it with liberality. Where I have differed with my contemporaries I have frequently done so without any direct reference to them; and if I could have devised the means of explaining myself in an intelligible manner in all cases without it, it would have been peculiarly agreeable to me to have availed myself of it.

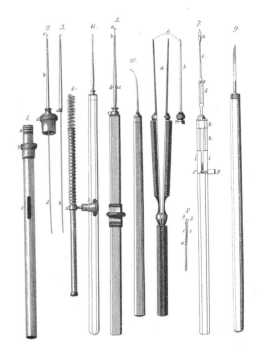

Figure 13.6 *Plate 5. Instruments for eye surgery designed by European surgeons (Langenbeck, Schlegintweit, Reisinger and Embden) (detailed descriptions are included)*

Finally, he wrote in a statement typical of Guthrie:

> That there are a great many surgeons in Europe, there are but few good operators, and principally for want of opportunity. If he cannot operate well himself he may still, by a knowledge of disease, prevent the necessity of its being done by others.

Contents

The book includes the treatment of inversion and eversion of the eyelids, pterygium, injuries to the eyeball and the removal of foreign bodies, the differential diagnosis of glaucoma and cataract, tumours within the orbit, and the causes, classification and diagnosis of cataract, together with a detailed description of its treatment by displacement of the lens anterior or posterior to the iris ('couching') or extraction of the lens. Also included is an interesting and detailed description of excision of the eyeball (first carried out in 1747 by the French surgeon Daviel).

Over 200 pages are devoted to *cataract*. The type of operation performed by Greek, Roman, Hindu and Arabic surgeons, the distinction between mature, immature, hard and soft cataract, when to operate if one or both eyes are affected, and the different techniques for the operation are all described and discussed. The 'couching' operation for cataract was considered by Guthrie to be 'infinitely shorter than that of extraction, requiring less apparent care in its performance and less manual dexterity'. However, Guthrie preferred extraction of the lens and, after describing the history of this procedure, he describes in detail his own technique, together with the post-operative care and problems associated with the operation. He also describes the techniques of European surgeons for this operation (Scarpa, Willbey, Beer and others). Operations for the division (or breaking up) of a cataract, either anterior or posterior to the iris, are discussed and described. A graphic and detailed description of a cataract extraction carried out in Calcutta in 1816 is interesting. Guthrie was one of the first surgeons to describe a congenital cataract.

Many case histories are incorporated into the text, as always in Guthrie's writings, and these add greatly to the narrative. Finally, surgical instruments for eye surgery are illustrated and described.

Incorporated into this book is Guthrie's *Treatise on the Formation of an Artificial Pupil,* previously published in 1819 (see Chapter 12). This occupies 125 pages. It was an operation for which he was well known and which he had used extensively. Sixty-nine of these pages review European surgeons' experience of this procedure.

CHAPTER 14

Hunterian Oration (1829)

This Oration[1] was delivered at the Royal College of Surgeons on 15th February 1830 and in it Guthrie acknowledged the debt that surgery owed to John Hunter's original research no fewer than 12 times. It was said to be memorable and was delivered 'fluently without notes, as afterwards had been done by Sir James Paget, Savory, Henry Power, Butlin and Moynihan'.[2] Further comments by a member of the audience present at the lecture are included in Chapter 5, p. 85.

A preliminary eulogy of John Hunter, in particular referring to his operation for popliteal aneurysm, is followed by the studies of Abernethy and Astley Cooper on iliac and carotid artery ligation, Guthrie's own pioneering operation of removal of the head of the humerus, the anatomy of the brain and its influence on the treatment of head injuries, the research of Cline and Astley Cooper on hernia, the recognition of dislocation of the hip joint, the work of Percival Pott on spinal disease, and finally the treatment of blindness.

We are assembled on this present occasion to commemorate the Anniversary of the birth of the late John Hunter, not in sorrow, not in sadness, nor with lamentations, but with a grateful remembrance of the inestimable services he rendered to mankind. We owe this opportunity to the munificent spirit of the late Dr Baillie and the present Sir Everard Home; interested it is true by the ties of relationship which existed between them but induced, I am satisfied, by a far more honourable feeling, that of holding him up to future observers both as a man indubitably possessed of the highest merit and as one who, by his virtue, his perseverance, his laborious, continued and unceasing exertions for the improvement of science, and the advancement of his art, had rendered services of the utmost importance to the first interests of society. I am satisfied that they had yet a nobler motive; that the comparison of his various excellencies might stimulate the bosoms of some that are yet unborn, might present them with inducements to equal, if possible, to excel him; that thus, whilst we pay due honours to the departed dead, we may accomplish that which would be the dearest wish of his heart if he were amongst us – be useful to the living.

The eight hundred pounds which those gentlemen each devoted to this special purpose, and the interest which is allotted to defray the expenses of this occasion, will purchase for them a far greater perpetuity of fame than they could have obtained by thrice the expenditure in any other way. Posterity, I am sure, will do them justice, and in their history and character there will be no part more bright than the record of the devotedness, the zeal, the disinterestedness in the cause of science, which they evinced on this occasion.

Mr Hunter was a man of singular aptitude for labour; unwearied in his researches after truth; a close observer and a steady reasoner, little addicted to theory, and that little only when founded upon the closest investigations of the operations of nature. I claim not for him the attributes of a superlative genius. He was a man like many amongst you; if there was one point – if there was one quality in which he was pre-eminent, it was that of perseverance; that quality he possessed in a peculiar degree; add to this that he was just and honest in all his dealings, and you have the character of the late John Hunter, and also of one of the noblest works of God.

Mr Hunter's object in the improvement of our science was to collect from every quarter of the globe such animals, such specimens as might show a particular mode of organisation, that by comparing them one with another he might be enabled to estimate their peculiar functions; and by going from the simplest to the most complex, he might understand that mechanism which was the most difficult to assess. He did more; he sought for those structures when in a seat of disease, that he might understand the peculiar derangement of function which accompanies them in that condition. Thus was he able, from a knowledge of anatomy, to lay the solid foundation upon which the superstructure of Physiology and Surgery was afterwards erected, which has raised his name in the opinion of the world to the high station that it has obtained.

The Museum which is contained within the walls of this College is not to be estimated according to the feelings of the present day. It is more than fifty years since he began to collect it; the facilities of communication that exist at the present moment were not then to be obtained. Countries which are now, as it were, at our own doors, were then distant journeys of months; the expense of the collection then was very different to what it would be at this moment, and yet there are few things which are now acknowledged to be scarce that are not to be found in the Museum at this moment. When we consider that this is the work of one individual, and that the assistance that he received was comparatively trifling, we must acknowledge that it is one of stupendous magnitude; it was not formed without the greatest labour; he spent his whole time, the better part of his life and, in addition to that, what few would devote, the whole of his fortune upon its formation. Mr Hunter died poor; but he left behind him riches which, I trust, through the exertions of this College, will raise for him a monument that will be imperishable.

It is not for its superficial beauties alone that the Museum is to be admired; it is necessary that it be searched into; it is necessary that its hidden treasures should be exposed; it is absolutely requisite that, in order to understand its value, every point should be set out and then the feelings, the conceptions of its founder, may be readily illustrated and developed.

There has been the greatest possible difficulty in arranging this collection, from the circumstances of the manuscripts which were connected with the individual articles having been either lost on the one hand, or destroyed under an erroneous feeling on the other. This has added greatly – immeasurably I may say – to the difficulties that have been experienced in forming a proper catalogue. The evils and difficulties which this entailed are on the eve of being overcome. The gentlemen, who for years have laboured to accomplish this great object, are on the point of finding all their wishes realised. That part of the catalogue which relates to the natural history is almost ready for the press; the osteological part of it is in a similar situation; and all that relates to the morbid anatomy is almost completely printed and ready to be submitted to the inspection of the public.

There is yet more wanted. It has been my lot, in the course of the last year, in searching through the museum for the purposes of the lectures which I had the honour to deliver in this place, to be able to estimate the value of a particular part of it. I came to that research acquainted with the opinions of the last thirty years – of those years which have passed since the death of Mr Hunter; and I found to my surprise that he had anticipated in the formation of this collection nearly the whole of those opinions. He had done more. He had laid a foundation that would allow me to refute a number of statements which certainly were untenable, and to the correctness of which many of our greatest continental writers have assented, that such and such diseases could not exist because the means did not exist which would admit of the formation of such diseases. As if to show the littleness of our knowledge of nature; as if to show how very little we knew of what he could perform, I have found in the history of the museum of Mr John Hunter, not only that such diseases could take place, but that they did take place in those very situations in which they said they could not occur. Our neighbours on the continent, whenever they have anything of this novel nature before them, do not lose an opportunity of submitting it to the public. They are well aware that the contents of a museum are perishable. They know well that even the house which holds it must in the course of time be shortly brought to the ground; they therefore take the means which will preserve to posterity those benefits which are of the greatest importance; and I should have been delighted to have done thus much in the book I am now publishing containing the observations I delivered here last year. I should have been delighted to have included those engravings in that book which would have illustrated the subjects on which I spoke; but I felt that in thus associating my own name with that of Hunter I should have been obtaining surreptitiously an honour that could not belong to me. I knew the permission that I had in this College to make drawings; that permission has been refused to no individual. Every individual has been permitted to take drawings of any article in the museum, with the simple restriction that, on the face of it, it be declared to have been copied from the museum of the College of Surgeons. There was never but one instance in which permission was refused; and then it was not when the request was made to illustrate a particular subject but where leave was asked to take drawings of the whole museum for mercenary motives and then the Board of Curators gave their refusal.

I say I should have been delighted to have expended my two or three hundred pounds in associating my name with that of Hunter and in transmitting it to posterity; but I felt that Government, which had purchased this museum and delivered it into the hands of the Council, had deposited with them a public trust; and that in taking advantage of a private opportunity I should have betrayed the permission granted to me by my colleagues. The labours of Mr Hunter will be exhibited and made known by the public act of this great body. It remains then with the Council to do that which shall enable us to say, in the language of the Roman poet 'His monument shall be more durable than brass'; that when this house shall be no more the public libraries of Europe shall still hand down his name to posterity with redoubled honours.

I am desirous not only of fulfilling the duties allotted to me in this oration – I am desirous of not only doing that which its founders have desired – but I should like to do that which would be agreeable to Mr Hunter if it were permitted to him for a moment to look down upon this sublunary space. I am sure he would say 'It is not by the praises you can bestow on me that I am to be propitiated; it is not by homage of that nature; the only offering I should wish to receive of you will be the record of the improvements you have made since I was taken from among you'. I shall endeavour, then, to do that which I think at the present moment would be agreeable to Mr Hunter if he were permitted to be a judge of our proceedings.

The subject which I had the honour to select last year for discussion before you was one in which Mr Hunter's character has shone forth with paramount industry and talent. His name is attached to an operation upon the arteries and to one which has laid the foundation for a great deal of – I may say for all – the improvement which has taken place in the several branches of our science up to the present moment.

Previous to Hunter's time that enlargement of a great artery which is denominated an aneurysm was a most fatal complaint. No operation was performed for it higher than the ham, except in one or two particular instances in which it had been attempted in the thigh. When this operation was performed according to the ancient method, in the ham, it was found to be attended with but very little success. The patient underwent the greatest possible danger and if he recovered at all it was only with a partial use of the extremity – it was usually with a useless limb; and this was so well known that that one of the contemporaries of Mr Hunter, just before he brought forward his improvement of the operation, considered the case to be so serious and so dangerous, that he declared it was better to amputate the limb than to perform the ancient operation. Mr Hunter, from the close investigations he was making which I have described to you, saw that the error consisted in performing the operation on the diseased part; and he was led to believe that if it were done at a certain distance from the part diseased, all the evils which happened would be avoided. He had carefully watched the progress of the cure by the simple operation of Nature alone. He saw that she filled the enlargement or sac with coagulated blood and that the cure afterwards proceeded to its termination favourably. The close reasoning which he was accustomed to exercise induced him to think that if he imitated this process he could not fail to meet with similar success. He did imitate it; he succeeded; not, indeed, in the first instance but he attempted it again as if satisfied that success would ensue; and I shall have occasion to point out to you presently the similarity of a series of circumstances which followed that success and by which he laid the foundation for all the beneficial results which have attended the brilliant operations since introduced into surgery.

We were not content to rest satisfied with leaving undone that which our ancestors could not do. It was said that an artery could have no ligature placed upon it unless the circulation through it was previously stopped; all the vessels, therefore, in the neighbourhood of the head and in the upper part of the body were abandoned to the operations of Nature, and when disease in them occurred death was the result. It was reserved for one of Mr Hunter's pupils – one of the most earnest, the most scientific followers of his example to do away with this difficulty. Mr Abernethy, called upon by the urgency of the moment, relying on the anatomical knowledge he possessed and which can scarcely be thoroughly possessed unless by one who is constantly in the habit of teaching and exercising his knowledge of those subjects – called upon by the urgency of the case, suddenly placed a ligature on the iliac artery – upon one iliac artery. The operation was unsuccessful. It was supposed the operation could not be made with success. Like his master he was not to be cast down; he tried the operation again and then Nature did not fail to reward his efforts. By the result of his first effort he was not deterred; but on repeating the operation in a similar manner it was crowned with success.

The arteries in the upper part of the body had been abandoned, as I have already said, to Nature. Here, again, the difficulties were not less ingeniously defeated by Sir Astley

Cooper who was the first to apply a ligature on the carotid artery; this was followed by a similar want of success. A second operation was performed which succeeded and established that operation as a proper operation – as an operation proper to be performed, and it is one which has since been performed and has been followed with the same success. We now even tie those arteries which are of the greatest importance within a few inches of the heart itself and in the operation look for recovery. Even the great trunk leading from the heart itself has been tied; and although in both instances in which it has been done – once by Sir Astley Cooper and once by Mr James of Exeter – success has not yet crowned the efforts that were made; but it is possible these may be the only instances in which it may be wanting.

There is another disease of these great vessels which is not, perhaps, at first quite so dangerous but which ultimately leads to as unfortunate results. It is where the vessel, the great artery itself, is not alone affected. But where a multiplicity of smaller vessels are found taking on an irregular, an extraordinary action, producing a disease which is equally unmanageable and which extends over a considerable surface. It was found difficult to submit this to any surgical operation; but the talents of Mr Hunter's successors have overcome it. We find that ligatures have been applied around these masses of disease with the most essential advantage. Sir Anthony Carlisle, Mr Lynn, Mr Lawrence, Mr White have given examples of the cure of such diseases. But the operation has even been carried further, where those vessels were so enlarged in size as almost to form an unmanageable disease from being composed of a series of vessels equal to the largest arteries; and where the ligature could not be placed around the mass, the enquiries of surgeons have found means of overcoming the difficulty. Thus a ligature, when no longer being capable of being placed around them, is carried through them from one side to the other, and by this division of the mass, though it could not be compressed by one ligature, a complete cure has been effected. For this particular improvement in the management of diseased arteries we are principally indebted to Mr Keate and Mr Brodie *[possibly an arteriovenous fistula]*.

In the time of Mr Hunter the operation of amputation was looked upon in a very different light to what it is at the present moment. Operations of the thigh were performed with considerable doubts and oftentimes with considerable

fears. It is within my own recollection that some operations, more severe than these, were considered hardly fair
and proper to be performed on the human body. It is not
often within the circle of civil life that some of the great
operations, such as amputation at the shoulder or at the
hip – the taking away the quarter of a man's body – are
rendered necessary; but in military surgery it has not been
uncommon on urgent occasions, occasions on which it
was not only a necessary thing but on which the surgeons,
having to decide at the moment, were called upon to act;
and called upon in this manner they were not found
wanting in their duty. The result has been that those operations which were at one time almost considered barbarous
and unfit to be performed are now done by all, done by
everybody, and with comparatively little consideration
when viewed with what was considered necessary thirty
years ago. We find that they have been crowned with
success. The operation of amputation at the hip joint has
been performed some four or five times; that is it has been
performed that number of times successfully among a
number of failures. I may say of this, as of some of the
preceding operations, in the words of a late author, that it
is 'a victory obtained by surgery over death'.

Mutilation, however, is a subject that can give us little
pleasure. It is a greater triumph to think that those cases
which twenty of thirty years ago were considered proper
subjects for amputation, have, by the improvements made
since the death of Mr Hunter, been saved without it. We
are often now capable of saving a limb when the head of
the extremity of the bone has been injured. Such, for
instance, as those that form the shoulder, the elbow and
the knee joints. Improved surgery has introduced the
practice of removing the extremities of the bones themselves and leaving the remainder of the bones to their fate;
and in a great number of instances where amputation of
the upper extremity would formerly have been performed,
the rounded head, the upper end of the humerus, which
moves in its socket, has been taken away and the arm has
been saved, giving to the patient a limb sufficiently useful
for all the essential purposes of future life. This, then, is the
triumph of improved surgery which is deserving of our
greatest praise – that it is often no longer necessary to
subject an individual to the most severe mutilations but
that it provides for the recovery of an individual with the
least possible loss to which the nature of the injury can
have subjected him.

These operations have all been performed with an ease and with a facility which in former days were unknown; and the reason is that the dread of haemorrhage from the great vessels which formerly occupied the minds of men is no longer experienced. The first step to this improvement was made by Mr Hunter when he placed a ligature on the middle of the thigh. He made the advance which was subsequently followed by Mr Abernethy and by Sir Astley Cooper in placing ligatures on the arteries of the upper parts of the body. When this was once done men were no longer filled with fearful apprehensions. The success which followed the repeated improvements induced persons to consider those operations, though they appeared horrible and dangerous, to be, when thoroughly investigated, really but small sources of dread; and this arising from the improved surgical treatment of the arteries. The fears that formerly existed have ceased any longer to take effect on the mind, and the operations now considered to be of the most common kind were, forty or fifty years back, regarded as the greatest and most serious. This is an improvement which I have no hesitation in saying we owe to the energies, the investigations and the reasonings of Mr Hunter.

There is another branch of surgery connected with anatomy upon which I should wish also to occupy your attention for a very few minutes. It is that which has relation to injuries of the head. In the time of Mr Hunter the anatomy of the brain was investigated after a peculiar fashion. The head was opened and the brain was sliced; it was cut away by portions; and, as parts came into view, or as they happened to be formed by the knife of the anatomist, so were they designated and named. But little was gained from this method of investigation. Very little knowledge indeed was acquired from it. It was a point that seemed to be stationary. During the last forty years great improvements indeed have taken place on this subject. The anatomy of the brain has ceased, in a great degree, to be examined in the manner I have pointed out. It has been taken out of the cranium and has been hardened by peculiar means which anatomists possess. They have been enabled in this way to trace those fibres which pass into it upwards and downwards; to trace the connections of one part with another; and the most important improvements have consequently taken place in the treatment of disease about these parts. Gall and Spurzheim did much in this enquiry, Reil did more. It is not, however, my intention to trespass on your time by stating that which has been done by foreign anatomists. I shall contents myself with saying that the greatest improvements that have taken place in this country have been effected by Mr Bell and by my excellent colleague and professor of anatomy Mr Mayo. They have shown that all the nerves of the body are not nerves capable of performing every function but that most of them, and indeed, each of them, have their respective duties; that some are nerves of motion, that some are nerves of sensation, that some are nerves of both; and in consequence of these beautiful discoveries we are enabled to treat those diseases which we formerly considered as doubtful, and dependant on chance and accident – we are now oftentimes enabled to treat them by operations leading to their complete cure. It is not on this point alone that mankind have to thank the exertions of those who seemed to preside in some degree over the evils which befall humanity; because with respect to the injuries of the head itself it was formerly the practice, the moment a man was cut on the head, to scalp him; if he was injured a little more he was sure of being trepanned. A man had no chance of escape from an injury of the head without an operation being performed by which he lost a considerable proportion of his skull and which of itself was likely to be attended with important consequences. But modern surgery, following the close system of investigation that was laid down by Mr Hunter after a more accurate research upon this point, has brought us now to regard the correct practice as almost essentially the reverse of what it formerly was. Thus the removal of a portion of the head for injuries not particularly serious and which was attended with more serious consequences even than even the accident itself, has been almost entirely abandoned. We undertake the treatment of these cases according to the symptoms which modern surgery has investigated, and the result has been a considerable saving of human life. On this point surgery deserves the warmest thanks it can obtain from the public at large.

There are other points which rise up before me possessing considerable and equal advantages; there are many of them showing even greater improvements than those I have noticed to you. If I refer to one single circumstance – if I refer to that disease which formerly used to be so much dreaded – hernia or rupture, I shall then bring to your recollection and show you at a glance the great improvements that have taken place. This class of injuries was considered to depend upon almost one cause alone; it was scarcely supposed that there were the differences amongst them that are now known to exist. The anatomy of the parts in which they occurred was by no means understood; it had never been clearly and thoroughly explained. We owe it to the last thirty years that we possess that clear and distinct understanding upon this point which enables those who have almost never seen the operation performed – yet following strict advice which is laid down for them following the remarks which are placed before them whilst students – they are enabled to perform the operation themselves and to perform it with success. We owe this to the united labours of several individuals. Mr Cline, in the first instance, pointed out a dissimilarity between two ruptures coming apparently from the same place, an error in the distinction of which might be followed by the most serious consequences; an error in distinguishing them which might be attended by the result, that in one case a great artery that would be lying on the one side might be divided whilst in the other case it would be found on the opposite side; so that if the method of operation usually in force had been adopted, it is more than probable in those days that the life of the patient would have been sacrificed. This observation, made first I say by Mr Cline, connected with an earnest desire for the improvement of the art to which he belonged, induced Sir Astley Cooper to investigate the point closely and the result was the discovery of new parts which had hitherto not been described and of new parts connected with this disease and the manner of performing the operation now generally adopted. It is in your recollection that the fascia which covers the lower part of the belly was, from its strength, distinguished by him from the common cellular structure with which it had previously been confounded. He not only did this but he illustrated those opinions which his master Mr Cline, had previously expressed; and he pointed out one rule which, if followed, would answer in every case of injury of this kind and would prevent the disastrous result which would inevitably follow such a mistake as that to which I have alluded. Instead of adopting the ancient practice of making the incision obliquely outwards, he gives you the distinct rule to make the incision directly upwards in either case and then all danger will be avoided.

The enquiry into the anatomy of hernia has been followed by others with great advantage. We certainly owe to foreign authors many improvements which I shall not now take up your time in going over. I shall only repeat that those operations which were formerly regarded as so dreadful that but few would venture to perform them, the consequence of which was that an immense number of persons lost their lives, have now, from the new lights of anatomical knowledge, become so easy, so satisfactory to the feelings of those who have to perform them that there is scarcely an individual to be found whose life is now lost without an operation having been performed upon him, or through a want of that care which would be afforded by an accomplished surgeon.

There are other points that I will endeavour to bring before you as concisely as I can. The subject of dislocations was one, in former days of considerable difficulty. Many of them were hardly known to take place at all. It is a very curious circumstance that a surgeon of the great hospital of St Thomas's should, until a few years back, have said that he had never seen a dislocation of the hip joint, an accident which is now, I may say, comparatively so common. It cannot be that there is so great a difference now in the mercantile transactions of this town, between the labours going on in it, and that persons are now so engaged that they are rendered peculiarly liable to this accident, formerly so infrequent. It could not be owing to causes of this kind because we know that the accident often takes place from causes which cannot be accounted for. Sometimes it does not require, comparatively, great violence to occasion it. It is therefore but fair to infer that in former days those accidents took place as generally as they do at the present moment but that they were not detected in the same ready manner; that the persons who were the subjects of them passed their days in a state which was presumed to be irremediable, solely because those whose duty it was to make themselves acquainted with the nature of such injuries were incapable of detecting the accident; not probably because they were unwilling to inform themselves but because they had not the opportunity of doing so. In order that a man should be able to remedy those great accidents, in order to overcome the difficulties they present, it is not by a cursory knowledge of his practice that he will be able to do so but it is by that knowledge which can only arise from dissection, and from dissection with his own hand, of those parts connected with the displacements of which he is afterwards called upon to judge. When any of those great operations is to be performed it is not the time for the surgeon to go to enquiring after what will enable him to perform them; it is necessary for him to call up the stores of information that are within himself; he must work with his head at the time he works with his hands; the two must be one and indivisible. Unless he is able to unite those two qualities it is impossible he can do what the surgeon ought to; it is impossible that he can do that which the public have a right to expect from him.

There are many other diseases, Gentlemen, which yet demand our attention. Until the time of Mr Hunter you will find that diseases of the spine and the diseases of the joints occupied but little or no attention. It is true, a contemporary of Mr Hunter – Mr Pott, a surgeon possessing almost an equal degree of knowledge, a gentleman remarkable for his enquiries and writings and for his knowledge of literature – a gentleman who may, perhaps be considered in one point of view, as the rival of Mr Hunter – he paid to this subject particular attention. I have said a rival; but I would say one who was generous and noble in all his feelings, entertaining a rivalry, not on those little trifling things which occupy so much attention in the present day, but a rivalry for the improvement of knowledge; and I cannot but recommend gentlemen to follow, at the present moment, an example which I trust will never be abandoned by his successors. Mr Pott, to those particular diseases, paid great attention; he showed the precise nature of one of the diseases which affect the bones and he pointed out at the same time the means by which it might be remedied. At the same period of time all those affections which attacked the joints were considered to be almost of a similar nature; they were all included and classed together under the denomination of white swelling; they were treated by the same method – a method inconsistent with sound surgery because it was not founded upon an accurate knowledge of disease. It was reserved for his successors of the present day to make the proper distinctions; to separate the one disease from the other; to show their formation; to trace them in their courses; to distinguish their different tendencies; to find out an accurate treatment and, therefore, to lead to happier results. It is true there is much yet to be done – many things yet remain; and there is an ample field, unfortunately I may say, unfortunately for future observations; but I must here say that for the knowledge we do possess of those diseases we are indebted to Messrs Pott, Crowther, Copeland, Brodie and the successor of Mr Pott, the present Mr Earle.

There are many other complaints which ancient surgery had in some degree abandoned. I would bring before you at the present moment a view of the improvements that have been made in another class of disease – diseases of the utmost importance I may say to the welfare of mankind. Those diseases which deprive a man of all his energies – which deprive him of all his youth – which deprive him of all his expectations in future life and yet leave him strictly in a state of health but without the capacity of exercising his powers either for himself or for others; I mean those diseases which lead to blindness. There are in this country individuals who confine themselves to one, two or three branches of the profession and separate those branches entirely from the others; so that instead of any advancement being made in those departments, it becomes their interest to keep the knowledge they have acquired, concealed. We have a peculiar instance of this in the case of Ruysch, a Dutch surgeon who was particularly successful in the operation for the stone. He would never tell the manner in which he did it; and when he was asked by two of his pupils, Albinus and Heister, to inform them how he performed it, he answered them, '**You ask me to give away that which is my bread!**' Is there a surgeon of the present day who would give a similar answer to such an enquiry? I am proud to say there is not. But when there is secrecy and any peculiarity of practice that leads to, and in fact it is, gross empiricism. Within the last thirty years, then, those diseases have become an object of attention to medical men. We are indebted to the late Mr Sanders for the establishment of an institution in the city for the cure of the blind, or, I would rather say, for the acquirement of knowledge upon that point by medical men; for it has diffused among medical men that degree of knowledge which could not have been acquired by any other means. I can safely say, in the hands of scientific men, as much good can be done in this department of our science as in any other branch of it; and that he who goes forth in the world without possessing the same knowledge of those complaints which he has on the subjects of hernia, stone, the arteries and other points, has not attained the degree of knowledge he ought to have acquired.

Sir, the silent monitor on the table informs me I have already occupied too much of your time; time that ought to be occupied in other pursuits. This hour-glass has expended itself, whilst the obligation under which I felt myself to mention those gentlemen who have distinguished themselves in the advancement of science, has only half run its course. I have a long catalogue of these yet before me; I have a long list of names with which it would delight me to occupy you on the present occasion; but I feel it has not permitted me to do so. I hope, Sir, I have said at least enough to stimulate some of those who are now before us to continue in their endeavours for the improvement of this science. I look upon the dawn of surgery as only to have arisen. It was founded – I have no hesitation in saying it was brought to light by the late John Hunter. **He raised it from the degraded state in which it had been placed by the superstition of former times.** He brought it out of that condition and left it in the hands of those who, I have no doubt, will be the means of elevating it to its full meridian splendour. It is, however, for those who are to come after us to effect this object. We have seen others do much and do well; let us hope never to see surgery fall back into its former state; let us hope that the light which has arisen will not be like the Mirage that deceives the eastern traveller, by inducing him to suppose at one moment that he is not far distant from the object of his pursuit and then cast him into the lowest abyss of despair. I feel, Sir, that even far brighter days are reserved for surgery. I am aware that it is not for us each to equal Mr. Hunter; it cannot be expected that we should; but **no one knows of what he is capable until he makes the effort**. It has been well said by the Roman poet, and his words have been copied by one of the most highly-gifted historians and ablest statesmen at the commencement of his work, that **he who begins has gained half**. Let this feeling then, I would say, urge those who are to come after us to the performance of their utmost efforts; and if they do not attain the same rank with John Hunter they will, if they act justly and honestly towards mankind, in life be respected, and in death be regretted.

The emphasis is given by the author to illustrate Guthrie's philosophical attitude to life and his respect for John Hunter.

References

1. Hunterian oration. *Lancet* 1829–30; **1**: 691–8 (issue 338, 20 February 1830).
2. *Plarr's Lives of the Fellows*. Bristol: John Wright, 1930; **1**: 482–5.

CHAPTER 15

Wounds and Injuries of the Arteries of the Human Body *(1830)*

Wounds and Injuries of the Arteries of the Human Body (Figure 15.1) was published in 1830 (with a second edition in 1846) and is based on nine lectures given at the Royal College of Surgeons. It comprised 130 case reports, half of which had been treated by Guthrie himself and half by other surgeons from the United Kingdom, Europe and America. Some of the case reports had been published previously in medical journals, the references to which are included. The book comprised only 97 pages, but its collation and analysis of the detailed case histories provides a wealth of information on arterial injuries and reflects a very large experience.

It makes fascinating reading, with some cases making a remarkable recovery, but it is unfortunate that the print is so small. The case reports illustrate the type of injury sustained in the early 19th century.

This book and *Commentaries on the Surgery of the War* (see Chapter 11) were undoubtedly Guthrie's most important and influential works.

The book records the 'practice of the most celebrated surgeons in Europe and America, with the critical remarks of the author on each'; and it describes whether Guthrie considered the treatment was correct, incorrect or could have been improved. Most case histories are followed by a detailed discussion of their treatment. The book concludes with a discussion of the technique for ligature of major arteries, from the aorta to the distal branches in the arm and leg. There are no illustrations.

In the text Guthrie emphasizes the difference between Anel's immediately proximal ligation for an aneurysm (described in 1710[1]) and Hunter's more distant proximal ligation (described in 1785[2]). He also discusses the significance of a collateral circu-

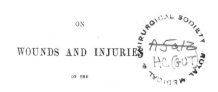

ON

WOUNDS AND INJURIES

OF THE

ARTERIES OF THE HUMAN BODY;

WITH THE

TREATMENT AND OPERATIONS

REQUIRED FOR THEIR CURE.

ILLUSTRATED BY 130 CASES, SELECTED FROM THE RECORDS OF THE PRACTICE OF
THE MOST CELEBRATED SURGEONS IN EUROPE AND AMERICA, WITH
THE CRITICAL REMARKS OF THE AUTHOR ON EACH.

BY G. J. GUTHRIE, F.R.S.

LONDON:

J. CHURCHILL, PRINCES STREET, SOHO.
HENRY RENSHAW, 356, STRAND.

1846.
[PRICE THREE SHILLINGS.]

Figure 15.1 *Title page of* Wounds and Injuries of the Arteries of the Human Body *(1846) (reproduced with permission from the Royal Society of Medicine, London)*

lation and stresses that this is only present in association with an aneurysm and *not* after an acute arterial injury.

An article based on these lectures was published in the *Edinburgh Medical and Surgical Journal.*[3]

Especially interesting and instructive cases are: cases 5–10 (complete division of a major artery), cases 13–16 (ligation of femoral artery, with survival of the leg), case 42 (traumatic aneurysm in lower leg), case 53 (Anel's operation for popliteal artery aneurysm), case 55 (subclavian artery ligation), case 56 (Anel's operation for axillary artery aneurysm), case 62 (temporary subclavian artery aneurysm), case 66 (infected axillary artery aneurysm), case 73 (subclavian artery ligation for axillary artery aneurysm), case 78 (blunt injury to axillary artery, with no external injury to arm), case 88 (post-operative haemorrhage after orchidectomy), case 91 (external iliac artery ligation), cases 94 and 100 ('useless external iliac artery ligation'), case 97 (external iliac artery ligation after sword wound), cases 106 and 107 (accidental incision of an aneurysm) and case 128 (control of haemorrhage from external carotid artery). Guthrie's 'conclusions' at the end of Lecture 1 and after case 31 (common iliac artery ligation) are revealing and informative.

It is interesting that in this book, published in 1830, 20th century American spelling was used for *haemorrhage* and *aneurysm* (i.e. *hemorrhage* and *aneurism*) – not present-day English spelling.

Preface

The Preface gives an indication of Guthrie's forthright style and dedication to surgery – and also his humanity and attitude to his work as a surgeon (see also Chapter 2, p. 23 and Chapter 18, p. 235).

> The following lectures are given for the purpose of showing the erroneous nature of the opinions entertained by many surgeons, even of the present day, with respect to the practice to be adopted in cases of Wounds and Injuries of Arteries; and with the view of demonstrating and firmly establishing the fact, that the practice recommended and generally pursued during the latter part of the war in Portugal, Spain, France and the Netherlands, is the only one which can be followed with safety and success. It will be a consolation to those who labour in the great work of diminishing the ills to which mankind is subjected, to know that some good has in this instance resulted from evil; that the knowledge which has been thus derived from one of the most sanguinary, distressing and eventful struggles recorded in modern history, is and will be pre-eminently useful in saving the lives of many for ages yet to come.

4, Berkeley Street, Berkeley Square
July 14th, 1846

Guthrie's policy for the treatment of arterial injury – a summary

Guthrie's 'general conclusions' are included at the end of Lecture 8 and the following is an abridged version:

1. The Hunterian operation for cure of an aneurysm is not applicable to the treatment of a wounded artery.
2. When a large artery is divided and bleeds the wound should be enlarged and a ligature placed on both the divided ends.
3. No operation should be performed on any artery unless it bleeds.
4. The intervention of muscle is not sufficient reason for ligating the artery at a distant point.
5. If the wound passes indirectly to the supposed arterial wound then a probe should be passed into the wound and an incision made to expose the injured artery.
6. Hand pressure is preferable to a tourniquet when operating on an aneurysm or a wounded artery.
7. The blood from the upper end of a divided artery is scarlet; that from the lower end is dark or venous in colour.

8. A flow of blood from the lower end of a divided artery is a favourable sign as it shows that the collateral circulation is probably sufficient to maintain the life of the extremity.

9. The collateral circulation is usually adequate if the axillary artery has been divided but not always in the case of the femoral artery.

10. The collateral circulation is almost always sufficient to maintain life in the extremity if the aneurysm has existed for 8–10 weeks.

11. If the femur has been broken and the femoral artery has been divided, amputation is usually necessary.

12. If a broken bone injures an artery and causes an aneurysm, the fracture must be treated first, and then the aneurysm later, after time has been given for a collateral circulation to be established to maintain the life of the limb.

13. Amputation is necessary forthwith if gangrene develops following an arterial injury.

14. After femoral artery and vein injury leading to gangrene of the foot, a below-knee amputation is preferable and less dangerous than a thigh amputation.

15. If gangrene of the lower leg develops, ceases, and then continues to extend, amputation is necessary as the gangrene will never cease to extend again.

Introductory lecture

Guthrie complained about the general lack of knowledge of the correct treatment for incised chest wounds or abdominal wounds. He also complained about the lack of profit from medical publishing; he himself had had to pay for the paper and printing of his books, and to provide a 10% commission to the printer and a 30% commission to the retailer for the sale of the book. Therefore, he preferred to publish his views on surgery in 'the weekly medical journals as may please to publish them'.

He considered the treatment of injured arteries was similarly not understood and that 'Mr Hunter's theory for the cure of diseased arteries' was not successful for the treatment of injured arteries. In his work as a surgical examiner he had found he was frequently acting as an instructor rather than an examiner and that consequently he 'was obliged to exercise a leniency when about to pronounce sentence of approval or rejection which often materially interferes with my sense of duty'.

The Peninsular War had led to a 'great improvement in the art and science of surgery in a degree which neither could, or would, have been effected' without the miseries of that war, and, as Sir Astley Cooper had said, 'that war had given to surgery its greatest impulse in the present century', a sentiment echoed by Sir Clifford Allbutt and Sir Gordon Taylor in the 20th century.[4,5] He emphasized how much his views on the treatment of injured limbs were very different from those of John Hunter, and that at that time he was 'not twenty nine years of age'. He noted that his views had now 'not only been generally adopted but pirated by some persons, and even advanced as something new by others many years' after he had published them.

He emphasized that the treatment of an arterial injury was very different from the treatment of an aneurysm and that the damaged artery must be ligated proximal *and distal* to the injury, unlike Hunter's treatment of an aneurysm, in which only proximal ligation was required.

His surgical experience in London during hospital and private practice over the last 30 years, 'during which he had enjoyed a share beyond his deserts', had confirmed his opinions gained during the Peninsular War.

Lecture 1: Aneurysm formation and complete arterial division

Ten case histories from the Peninsular War are described and summarized here.

British anatomists described three layers in an arterial wall – a strong external layer, a fibrous, pseudomuscular, contractile middle layer ('readily torn by a slight degree of extension') and a thin inner layer. Heller and Malgaine (both French anatomists) recognized a fourth layer between the inner and middle layers, which they thought to be the principal site of arterial disease.

Cases 1 and 2: Inadvertent injury to ulnar and axillary artery, controlled by firm pressure. A murmur over the artery gradually diminished and distal pulsation returned.

Case 3: Arrow injury in neck opposite carotid artery bifurcation, leading to an aneurysm which did not increase in size until death in action one year later. No post-mortem.

Case 4 (of Mr Keate at St George's Hospital): Arteriovenous aneurysm of femoral artery following a knife wound. Patient 'in bad health' and aneurysm therefore controlled by external pressure, which was thought to have led to a reduction in its size.

Cases 5–10: Six cases of complete division of an artery following severe battle injuries, in two of which a limb had been blown off; no haemorrhage had occurred in these two cases due to spasm of the torn artery. Haemorrhage from the distal end of the divided artery had occurred in two cases and from the proximal end in another two cases, all leading to a fatal outcome.

Three important lessons were learnt from the treatment of these injuries:

1. Arterial spasm can arrest haemorrhage, even from an artery as large as the femoral.
2. Haemorrhage from the distal end is venous in colour, though this is less marked in the axillary artery because of a better collateral circulation in the upper arm.
3. Haemorrhage from the distal end can be controlled by firm external pressure.

Lecture 2: Partial division of an artery

If the artery is only partially divided it can neither retract nor contract, and will continue to bleed 'until it destroys the patient or pressure can be accurately applied'.

Cases 11–12: Brachial and femoral artery ligated above and below the wound.

Cases 13–16: Incised wounds of femoral artery, in three of which an aneurysm developed one month later, and in one case 12 years later. In these four cases the artery was ligated above and below the injury, *with survival of the limb*. All four patients recovered.

Cases 17–19: Femoral and popliteal aneurysms – proximal arterial ligation. It was concluded that distal gangrene was more common after ligation for an arterial wound than after ligation for an aneurysm.

Cases 20–28: Injury to femoral and popliteal artery. In many of these cases the artery had been ligated, sometimes too late, and gangrene had developed.

Case 29: A woman who had developed lower leg gangrene and in whom the femoral artery up to the inguinal ligament was thick and hard. ? Cause. Above-knee amputation. Limb preserved in College museum.

Case 30: Blunt injury to popliteal artery leading to distal gangrene. Successful amputation performed.

Case 31: Ligation of common iliac artery for a gluteal swelling thought to be an aneurysm. Patient died one year later and post-mortem showed the ligation to be ⅝ inch distal to aortic bifur-cation and that a good collateral circulation had developed. Specimen in College museum.

Four conclusions were drawn from these cases:

1. Hunter's advice for proximal ligation for aneurysm is not applicable to recent traumatic aneurysm nor to haemor-rhage from an injured artery.
2. The extent of a collateral circulation depends upon the length of time since injury.
3. The collateral circulation is always capable of maintaining an adequate distal blood supply after an upper limb arterial injury but not always after a lower limb injury, unless a subsequent aneurysm has developed.
4. If the femoral vein has to be ligated as well as the artery, then gangrene will inevitably occur.

Case 32: Not described.

Case 33: Musket ball injury which fractured ulna. Brachial artery ligated due to haemorrhage from ulnar artery. Patient recovered.

Case 34: Similar to Case 33. Brachial artery torn and treated by proximal and distal ligation. Patient recovered.

Case 35: Musket ball injury to lower leg. Below-knee ampu-tation. Patient died.

Case 36: Similar injury to Case 35. Femoral artery ligated. Further haemorrhage led to amputation. Patient died.

Case 37: Musket ball injury in mid-thigh, leading to later aneurysm. Femoral artery ligated. Two weeks later infection led to amputation. Patient died.

Lecture 3: Effect of application of a ligature

The macroscopic and microscopic changes after arterial ligation are discussed. It was concluded that the ligature should be 'round and small, provided it be sufficiently strong'. An artery may be injured by external violence without being punctured.

Case 38: Musket ball injury – ball passed deep to the gluteus maximus. Haemorrhage controlled by external pressure. Two weeks later, after further repeated haemorrhages, wound explored and two branches of gluteal artery tied. Patient died two days later. ? Reason why. Post-mortem showed 'no adhesion had taken place. It is evident that operation should have been done in the first instance'.

Case 39 (of Mr Carmichael): Penetrating knife wound in hip leading to traumatic aneurysm of gluteal artery. After five days this increased in size. Proximal ligation of gluteal artery at its exit from ischiatic notch. Patient recovered.

Case 40 (of Prof. Baroni, Bologna): Gluteal artery injury. Abscess developed at site of wound – drained. Wound reopened later due to haemorrhage. Gluteal artery ligated. Patient recovered.

Case 41 (of Delpech, Montpellier): Injury to femoral artery by blunt trauma – artery ligated. Patient recovered.

Case 42 (of Baron Larrey): Lower leg wound led to aneurysm of ? anterior or ? posterior tibial artery, ? advise amputation. Femoral artery ligated and lower limb survived. Extensive discussion of the treatment of this patient follows, which Guthrie considered to be incorrect even though the patient survived.

Case 43: Fractured femur due to blunt injury. Aneurysm two weeks later in lower thigh and toes became black. Amputation advised but not carried out. Gangrene extended and patient died.

Case 44 (of Sir Anthony Carlisle): Ruptured popliteal aneurysm, which led to swelling of lower leg two weeks later. Femoral artery ligation advised by Guthrie but Carlisle laid open the lower leg, leading to uncontrollable haemorrhage. Amputation necessary and patient died.

Case 45 (of Astley Cooper): Similar to case 44.

Cases 46 and 47 (of Mr S. Cooper): Similar to case 44.

Case 48 (of Mr Stanley): Knife injury to peroneal artery. Patient died two weeks later from wound infection.

Case 49 (of Mr Stanley): Glass injury to posterior tibial artery. Proximal and distal ligation. Patient recovered.

Case 50: Musket ball injury to lower leg. Persisting haemorrhage for two weeks and therefore operation necessary. Detailed description of operation. Proximal and distal ligation of injured peroneal artery. Patient recovered.

Case 51 (of Mr Hall, East Retford): Patient thrown from his horse, leading to posterior tibial artery laceration. Haemorrhage partially controlled by tourniquet. Proximal and distal ligation. Patient recovered.

Case 52: Posterior tibial artery injury from a joiner's chisel. Proximal and distal ligation. Patient recovered.

Case 53: Below-knee amputation following compound fracture and dislocation of ankle joint. Three days later small bleeding aneurysm developed one inch above site of arterial ligation. Ligation of artery midway between aneurysm and its origin from the popliteal artery (the operation of Anel). Patient recovered.

Case 54: Fractured tibia and fibula due to musket ball injury, leading to infection. Secondary haemorrhage after one month. Proximal ligation of artery. Patient recovered. Discussion of technique of ligation of posterior tibial and peroneal arteries included.

Lecture 4: Wounds and injuries of the axillary artery

The axillary artery has not fared better in many instances than the posterior tibial and peroneal arteries. The same dread of dividing muscular fibres has overcome all other considerations.

Guthrie analysed the 69 operations reported by Norris of Pennsylvania in 1845, either above or below the clavicle – 36 recovered and 33 died.

Case 55: The first recorded case of ligature of the subclavian artery (by Mr Keate, Surgeon–General to the Forces) (no date given) for a ruptured axillary aneurysm following gunshot wound of some months' standing. He divided the pectoral muscle 'dipped down twice with a needle and thread and the second time secured the artery'. Patient recovered.

Comment: Guthrie added that he had 'since thought of the two dips of the surgeon's needle and had even ventured to think that the patient was as fortunate in his escape from his doctor as from his disease'. Guthrie had witnessed the operation but 'had been too young to know anything about the matter and too much in awe of the Surgeon–General to suppose for a moment that anything he did was wrong'.

Case 56 (of Mr Chamberlaine, Jamaica in 1814): Cutlass wound and 18 weeks later large axillary aneurysm developed. Subclavian artery ligated below clavicle (this was the operation of Anel, as opposed to Hunter's ligation at a distance from the aneurysm). Patient recovered.

Case 57: Musket ball injury to axillary artery. Patient died from haemorrhage before operation carried out.

Case 58: Sabre wound into axilla. Healed 'without difficulty'.

Case 59: Axillary artery injury. Pectoral muscles divided. Proximal and distal ligatures applied. Patient died from associated chest injury.

Case 60 (of Delpech, Montpellier): Brachial artery ligation. Patient died 10 days later from sepsis.

Case 61 (of Delpech's assistant): Subclavian artery ligation due to haemorrhage after shoulder joint amputation. Patient died on fifth day 'exhausted'.

Case 62 (of Baron Larrey): Sword wound above clavicle causing injury to subclavian artery and vein. Arm cold with no pulse. Aneurysm developed and subsided after 20 days, though thrill remained. Patient recovered. Four years later no pulse detectable in ulnar or radial arteries but arm was warm and viable.

Case 63 (of Delpech, Montpellier): Same injury and outcome as case 62.

Comment: These two cases show that large arteries should be 'left alone until they bleed. Formidable operations are not to be done on the speculation that they may be required and this should never be forgotten'.

Case 64 (of Baron Larrey): Ulnar artery injury leading to an aneurysm. Brachial artery ligated. Patient recovered.

Case 65 (of Catanoso, Messina): Severe haemorrhage after axillary artery injury. Artery ligated below clavicle. Infection led to secondary haemorrhage. Patient recovered.
    Comment: The artery should have been ligated proximally and distally.

Case 66 (of Montanini, Naples): Axillary artery aneurysm following injury. Axillary artery ligated below clavicle. Aneurysm suppurated and discharged pus but no bleeding occurred. Patient recovered.
    Comment: The axillary artery distal to aneurysm must have closed or patient would have bled to death.

Case 67 (of Mr Dupuytren): Axillary aneurysm similar to cases 55 and 56.

Case 68 (of Lalleland, Montpellier): Subclavian artery ligation above clavicle for axillary artery aneurysm due to sword wound. Infection in aneurysm – discharged pus. Radial pulse returned after one month. Patient recovered.

Case 69 (of Prof. Blasius, Halle, Germany): Armpit injury causing presumed injury to axillary artery and vein. Subclavian artery ligated below clavicle. Patient died two days later from further haemorrhage and post-mortem showed bleeding had been from adjacent collateral smaller arteries.

Case 70 (of Dr Monteath, Glasgow): Blunt injury to upper arm. Twelve days later abscess in upper arm drained, followed by haemorrhage. Axillary artery ligated. Patient recovered.

Case 71 (of Desault, Paris): Sword injury to axillary artery which was ligated. Patient died six days later from gangrene.

Case 72 (of Dr Segond, French Guiana): Aneurysm following wound to axillary artery. Subclavian artery ligated above clavicle. Patient recovered.

Case 73 (of Dr Nott, Alabama): Axillary artery aneurysm after gunshot wound to upper arm. Subclavian artery ligated above clavicle. Patient recovered.

Case 74 (of Mr White, USA): Same as case 73.

Case 75 (of Dr Buchanan, Glasgow): Injury to brachial artery. Subclavian artery ligated above clavicle. Patient died five days later from distal gangrene.
    Comment: The axillary artery should have been ligated below the clavicle to preserve the collateral circulation.

Case 76 (of Dr Gibson, Pennsylvania): Subclavian artery ligated above clavicle for axillary aneurysm. Patient died 23 days later from gangrene.

Case 77: Ruptured subclavian artery due to blunt trauma. Subclavian artery ligated. Patient recovered. Almost a year later radial artery pulsation returned.

Case 78 (of Mr Stanley): Injury to arm and thigh by a wagon wheel. No outward sign of injury to arm, which was cold and pulseless. Twenty-four hours later patient died. Post-mortem showed inner and middle coats of brachial artery to be 'completely divided'.

Case 79 (of Sir Charles Bell): 'A girl had her arm torn off by machinery.' Axillary artery ligated. Patient died later from haemorrhage due to collateral circulation, despite ligature of axillary artery.

Case 80 (of Dr Post, New York): Scythe injury causing division of axillary artery. Amputation two inches below shoulder joint. Three weeks later arterial haemorrhage required ligation of subclavian artery above clavicle. Patient recovered.

Case 81 (of M. Haspel): Injury to axillary artery by a sword in a duel. Severe haemorrhage. Subclavian artery ligated below clavicle. Gangrene of arm led to amputation. Patient died a few days later.

Case 82: Injury to brachial artery by a sword in a duel. Controlled by compression. Patient recovered.

Case 83 (of M. Haspel): Sword wound to brachial artery. Ligated. Patient recovered.

Case 84: Patient thrown out of a gig. Rupture of axillary artery led to a large haematoma. Continued bleeding occurred intermittently for next month, only partially controlled by pressure.

Subclavian artery ligation failed to arrest haemorrhage and therefore amputation at shoulder joint necessary. Patient recovered.

Case 85 (of Dr Mackenzie): Fall on to a red-hot poker which entered axilla and eight days later a large eschar separated, followed by severe haemorrhage. Subclavian artery ligated above clavicle. Patient recovered.

Case 86: Shell injury led to amputation of arm close to shoulder joint. Infection of stump caused haemorrhage and it was difficult to control bleeding artery below clavicle. Patient recovered. Extensive discussion of treatment is given.

Case 87 (of Dr Stanley): Femoral hernia operation. One hour after operation haemorrhage from wound, controlled by pressure. Patient died two days later from peritonitis. Post-mortem showed haemorrhage had occurred from branch of epigastric artery.

Case 88: Left orchidectomy. Post-operative haemorrhage occurred and the coagulated blood resembled intestine! Wound explored and haemorrhage seen to be from small artery 'in the integuments near the external ring. A single thread ligature settled the matter'.

Case 89 (of Mr Quain, University College Hospital): Penetrating wound of axilla. Six days later no radial pulse detected. Pulsation returned five days later. Patient recovered.

Lecture 5: Non-applicability of Hunter's operation if wounded artery cannot be seen

Case 90 (of Hadwin and Quain, Leicester): Ruptured popliteal aneurysm. Femoral artery ligated at margin of sartorius. Two weeks later haemorrhage occurred and femoral artery ligated below inguinal ligament. Leg amputated above the lower ligature as haemorrhage not controlled. Further haemorrhage from collateral vessels and external iliac artery ligated. Patient recovered.

Case 91: Musket ball injury to thigh three inches below inguinal ligament. Wound healed. Two months later aneurysm at site of wound. External iliac artery ligated. Patient died three days later from gangrene of leg.

    Comment: The collateral circulation had not had time to develop.

Case 92 (of Delpech, Montpellier): External iliac artery ligated for a similar injury to case 91. Patient died from gangrene of leg.

Case 93: Musket ball injury just below inguinal ligament. Two days later severe haemorrhage. External iliac artery ligated. Patient died from infection one week later.

Case 94 (of Dr Buchanan, Glasgow): Boy injured by wheel of a rail wagon. Eighteen days later severe haemorrhage occurred from groin and repeated twice. External iliac artery ligated and later (because of further haemorrhage) femoral and inguinal arteries ligated. Patient died from exhaustion due to large abscess on ilium and sacrum.

   Comment: The inguinal artery should have been ligated *immediately* above and below site of injury. The external iliac artery ligation was useless as it failed to prevent development of collateral circulation.

Case 95 (of Heaviside, Howship and Chevalier, London): Blunt injury to thigh below inguinal ligament. Incipient dry gangrene but amputation not carried out. Eighteen days later severe haemorrhage and external iliac artery ligated but haemorrhage continued. Therefore original wound reopened and lower end of femoral artery ligated. Haemorrhage ceased but patient died 'from exhaustion' several days later.

Case 96 (of Mr Norman): Pitchfork injury to upper thigh. Haemorrhage from wound gradually increased and one week later became very profuse. Wound opened but artery could not be identified. Therefore external iliac artery ligated. Haemorrhage not controlled and therefore femoral artery ligated. Gangrene of leg developed. Above-knee amputation. Patient recovered.

Case 97 (of M. Lutens, France): Sword wound to femoral artery. External iliac artery ligated but haemorrhage continued due to collateral circulation. Gangrene of leg. Patient died.

   Comment: The ligature must be applied close to actual arterial wound.

Case 98: Aneurysm following knife wound to upper third of thigh. Femoral artery ligated below inguinal ligament. Three weeks later further haemorrhage and external iliac artery ligated. Patient recovered.

Case 99 (of M. Jobert, Paris): Femoral artery ligated one inch below inguinal ligament following wound to femoral artery deep to sartorius, where there was an aneurysm. Patient died 17 days later from haemorrhage from end of ligated artery.

Case 100 (of Dr Portal, Palermo): Secondary haemorrhage following excision of enlarged glands in groin. External iliac artery ligated above epigastric artery. Haemorrhage continued and femoral artery and vein ligated. Patient died from peritonitis and gangrene caused by useless external iliac artery ligation.

Case 101 (of Dr Murray): Large aneurysm one year after blunt injury to thigh. Femoral artery ligated (Anel operation). Further severe haemorrhage. External iliac artery ligated. Patient recovered.

Case 102 (of Baron Dupuytren): Aneurysm after blunt injury to groin. External iliac artery ligated. Patient recovered.

Case 103 (quoted by Sir Charles Bell, and treated by another surgeon): Groin wound. Femoral artery ligated. Haemorrhage recurred and patient died. Therefore, said Bell, distal ligation also necessary.

Case 104: Ulcerated bubo in groin. External pubic artery involved in bubo and it burst. Repeated haemorrhages controlled by pressure and examination showed femoral artery also to be involved and bleeding. External iliac artery ligated. Two days later vesication developed in thigh. High amputation. Patient recovered.

Case 105 (of Dr Warren, Boston): Amputation of thigh due to 'disease of condyles of femur'. Haemorrhage two weeks later. Femoral artery ligated one inch below inguinal ligament proximal to profunda artery. Patient recovered.

Case 106: Accidental incision into aneurysm in lower thigh. Amputation. Patient died a few days later from 'a defect of constitution'.

Case 107: Aneurysm three inches below inguinal ligament. Opened by mistake. External iliac artery ligated. Patient died two days later from gangrene.

Case 108: Femoral artery aneurysm extending under inguinal ligament. External iliac artery ligated. Patient recovered.

Case 109 (of Dr Horner, Pennsylvania): Femoral artery aneurysm extending under inguinal ligament. External iliac artery ligated. Sac opened, leading to severe haemorrhage. Femoral artery ligated above and below aneurysm. Death from 'exhaustion' on sixth day.

   Comment: To open the aneurysmal sac was unnecessary.

Case 110 (of Dr Horner, Pennsylvania): Pistol ball injury in upper thigh, leading to aneurysm below inguinal ligament. Femoral artery ligated but four days later gangrene ('mortification') of leg developed. Amputation two weeks later. Patient died. ? Why.

Case 111 (of Dr Brainert, St Louis, USA): Aneurysm under inguinal ligament one year after fracture of neck of femur (due to arterial injury from broken bone). External iliac artery ligated. Patient recovered.

Case 112 (of B. Cooper): Compound fracture of femur, causing aneurysm four days later. Femoral artery ligated. Patient recovered.

Lecture 6: No operation should be done on a wounded artery unless it bleeds at the time when the ligature is applied

Case 113: Musket ball injury behind greater trochanter and track emerged on the inside of the anterior thigh. Severe haemorrhage several days later, controlled by a tourniquet. When tourniquet released no more haemorrhage. Further haemorrhage later controlled by pressure. Wound explored but artery did not bleed. Patient recovered.

Case 113 (of Baron Larrey) [case number repeated]: Sword injury to upper thigh – ? injury to femoral artery. Two days later pulsating swelling in groin but this subsided during the next three days.

Case 114 (of Mr Porter, Dublin): Knife injury to profunda artery in upper thigh. Bleeding controlled, restarted again a day later. Again controlled by pressure. Patient recovered.

Case 115 (of Mr Cock, Guy's Hospital): Knife injury to inner mid-thigh. Severe haemorrhage. Femoral artery ligated 'about mid-thigh'. Wound infection but eventual recovery.

Case 116 (of no named surgeon): Duckshot injury to upper thigh. Two weeks later limb very swollen. Healed entry wound incised, leading to severe haemorrhage. Controlled with difficulty by pressure. Patient died one week later.

Case 117: Wound of upper right thigh with exit wound in left groin. Haemorrhage controlled by pressure. External iliac artery ligated 10 days later. Patient died two days later. Post-mortem showed aneurysm of femoral artery.

Case 118 (of no named French surgeon): Scissors injury to armpit. Repeated haemorrhage 4th–8th days after injury. Subclavian artery ligated above clavicle. Infection of wound caused further haemorrhage. Innominate artery ligated. Patient died 10 hours after operation.

   Comment: Two principles are to be observed in cases of wounded arteries: (1) 'No operation should be performed on a wounded artery unless it bleeds'; and (2) 'No operation to be done for a wounded artery in the first instance but at the spot injured, unless such operation appears to be impractical'.

Lecture 7: Wounds and injuries of the throat and mouth implicating the carotid artery

Case 119: Fatal ulceration of the carotid arteries by a retained foreign body in oesophagus.

Case 120 (of Mr Collier): Sword injury to left jaw which entered the mouth and lacerated the tongue. Continued haemorrhage required ligation of common carotid artery. Patient recovered. No mention of possible hemiplegia.

Case 121 (of Mr Mayo, England): Haemorrhage from throat ulcer. Common carotid artery ligated. Patient recovered. No mention of possible hemiplegia.

Case 122 (of Mr Luke): Persisting haemorrhage from throat ulcer. Left carotid artery (presumably external) ligated. Patient recovered.

Case 123: Cut throat. Internal jugular vein injured. Ligated. Eight days later arterial haemorrhage and it was evident that carotid artery had also been injured. External carotid artery ligated. Patient died next day 'from weakness'.

Case 124: Penknife wound to throat. Common carotid artery ligated. Patient died later. No mention of possible hemiplegia.

Case 125 (of Mr Vincent): Right common carotid artery ligation for aneurysm, leading to a left hemiplegia and death six days later.

Case 126: Haemorrhage following a throat injury. Right common carotid artery ligated, resulting in a left hemiplegia. Patient died six days later.

Case 127 (of Prof. Sedillot): Knife injury to right jaw below ear. External carotid artery ligated but haemorrhage continued. A few days later infection developed in knife wound. Common carotid artery ligated, leading to hemiplegia and death 10 days later.

Case 128 (of Dr Twitchell, USA): Severe gunshot wound to mouth and pharynx. Ten days later severe haemorrhage from exposed external carotid artery. Common carotid artery ligated below its bifurcation but haemorrhage persisted. Haemorrhage controlled by continued pressure on artery 'against base of skull'. Patient recovered. [This is a remarkable case report – how fortunate was the patient!]

Case 129 (of Dr Warren, Boston, USA): Left carotid artery ligated for 'an erectile tumour of lower lip'. One month later right carotid artery ligated. Patient recovered. ['Carotid artery' in text – presumably external.]

Lecture 8

The precise, detailed technique for ligation of aorta, iliac, internal and external iliac, gluteal, sciatic and femoral arteries is described.

Lecture 9

The precise, detailed technique for ligation of posterior tibial, peroneal, tibial, carotid, innominate, subclavian, brachial, ulnar and radial arteries is described.

References

1. de Moulin D. Dominique Anel and his operation for aneurysm. *Bull Hist Med* 1960; **34**: 498–507.

2. Power D'Arcy. Hunter's operation for cure of aneurysm. *Br J Surg* 1929; **17**: 196.

3. On the diseases and injuries of the arteries. *Edinburgh Med Surg J* 1830; **34**: 349–70.

4. Allbutt TC. *The Historical Relations of Medicine and Surgery*. London: MacMillan, 1905.

5. Gordon-Taylor G. The thoracic injuries of war. *Br J Surg* (War Surgery Suppl.) 1952; **3**: 381.

CHAPTER 16

Memoir on the Treatment of Venereal Disease without Mercury *(1830)*

G uthrie was opposed to the use of mercury for the treatment of venereal disease because of the unfortunate side effects which he had seen in the civilian hospitals in Lisbon during the Peninsular War. In 1830 the French *Memoir on the Treatment of Venereal Diseases without Mercury* by Desruelles described the treatment employed at the Val-de-Grâce military hospital in Paris and included 33 pages concerning the observations of Guthrie on this treatment (Figure 16.1).

Guthrie wrote:

> There are no diseases to which the male sex is so very obnoxious *[sic]* as those of the sexual organs, and there are none which have more occupied the attention of surgeons; yet there is not a subject in surgery of equal importance on which less has been written since the time of Mr Hunter

and he hoped his observations 'would elucidate a subject beset with so many difficulties; but the more I consider in which way this may be accomplished, the greater I find the obstacles to be surmounted'.

At the York Hospital in Chelsea Guthrie had treated 1084 cases of primary syphilis, 386 with mercury and 698 without mercury. There appeared to be no difference in the efficacy of this treatment, either on the primary chancre or in the incidence of the later secondary symptoms, and as a result of this investigation James McGrigor issued an army memorandum in 1819 which advocated Guthrie's regime; the treatment was by 'mild means, that is by dry lint, ointment and lotions, for the most part not containing mercury', together with potassium iodide. The treatment also included the use of purgatives, 'an emollient and soothing application of cold or warm water, sometimes

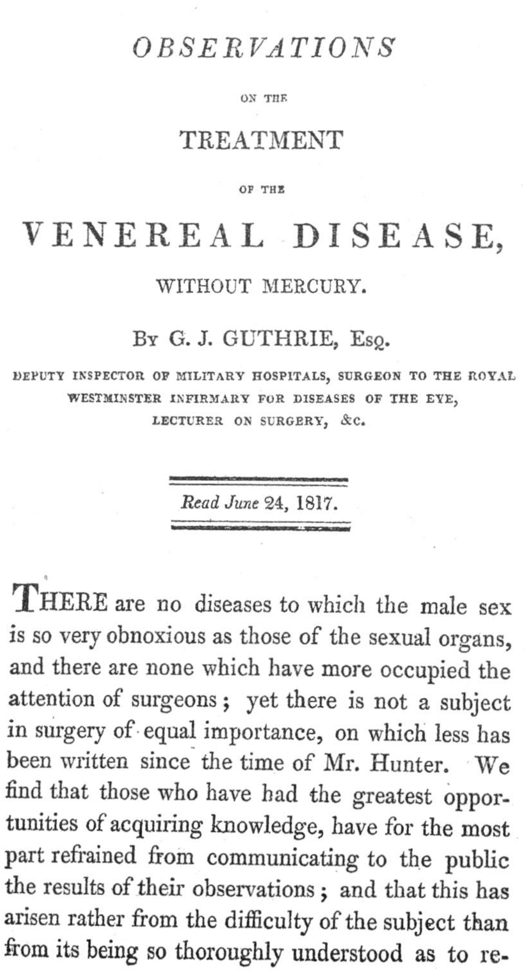

OBSERVATIONS

_{ON THE}

TREATMENT

_{OF THE}

VENEREAL DISEASE,

WITHOUT MERCURY.

BY G. J. GUTHRIE, ESQ.

<sub>DEPUTY INSPECTOR OF MILITARY HOSPITALS, SURGEON TO THE ROYAL
WESTMINSTER INFIRMARY FOR DISEASES OF THE EYE,
LECTURER ON SURGERY, &c.</sub>

Read June 24, 1817.

THERE are no diseases to which the male sex is so very obnoxious as those of the sexual organs, and there are none which have more occupied the attention of surgeons ; yet there is not a subject in surgery of equal importance, on which less has been written since the time of Mr. Hunter. We find that those who have had the greatest opportunities of acquiring knowledge, have for the most part refrained from communicating to the public the results of their observations ; and that this has arisen rather from the difficulty of the subject than from its being so thoroughly understood as to re-

mixed with *liquor plumbi or cupri* (lead or copper) and a nitro-muriatic acid bath'. The efficacy of this treatment was confirmed at various army hospitals in Europe, including the Val-de-Grâce in Paris.

Figure 16.1 *Title page of* Observations on the Treatment of Venereal Disease without Mercury *by Guthrie which was incorporated in Desruelles'* Memoir *(reproduced with permission from the Royal Society of Medicine, London)*

CHAPTER 17

Extraction of a Cataract from the Human Eye *(1834)*

Extraction of a Cataract from the Human Eye (Figure 17.1) was published in 1834 and sold for the benefit of the Royal Westminster Eye Hospital. Guthrie thought that previously published descriptions of the operation were not precise enough and did not adequately describe how to avoid the problems which might be encountered. He thought that surgeons who had described the operation 'did not quite tell all' in their publications, either intentionally or unintentionally, and he hoped that this short book of 44 pages would correct this. There were no illustrations.

A description of hard and soft cataract was followed by a description of how to examine the eye and whether or not both eyes should be operated on at the same session. The extraction of a hard cataract (extraction was not applicable to a soft cataract) was described in great detail. The technique for operation had changed since his previous book on this subject was published in 1823, when the operator sat in front of the patient; now it was advised that the surgeon should stand behind the patient.

A 12–16 oz venesection was advised after operation to prevent inflammation; if this should occur the application of leeches to the forehead was advised.

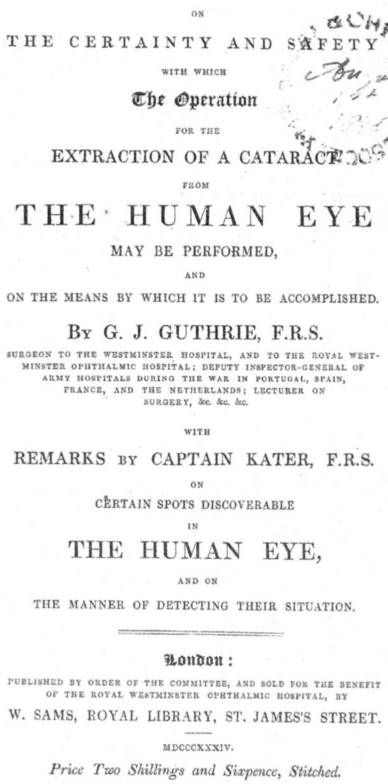

Figure 17.1 *Title page of* Extraction of a Cataract from the Human Eye, *published in 1834 (reproduced with permission from the Royal Society of Medicine, London)*

ON

THE CERTAINTY AND SAFETY

WITH WHICH

𝕿𝖍𝖊 𝕺𝖕𝖊𝖗𝖆𝖙𝖎𝖔𝖓

FOR THE

EXTRACTION OF A CATARACT

FROM

THE·HUMAN EYE

MAY BE PERFORMED,

AND

ON THE MEANS BY WHICH IT IS TO BE ACCOMPLISHED.

By G. J. GUTHRIE, F.R.S.

SURGEON TO THE WESTMINSTER HOSPITAL, AND TO THE ROYAL WEST-
MINSTER OPHTHALMIC HOSPITAL; DEPUTY INSPECTOR-GENERAL OF
ARMY HOSPITALS DURING THE WAR IN PORTUGAL, SPAIN,
FRANCE, AND THE NETHERLANDS; LECTURER ON
SURGERY, &c. &c. &c.

WITH

REMARKS BY CAPTAIN KATER, F.R.S.

ON

CERTAIN SPOTS DISCOVERABLE

IN

THE HUMAN EYE,

AND ON

THE MANNER OF DETECTING THEIR SITUATION.

𝕷𝖔𝖓𝖉𝖔𝖓 :

PUBLISHED BY ORDER OF THE COMMITTEE, AND SOLD FOR THE BENEFIT
OF THE ROYAL WESTMINSTER OPHTHALMIC HOSPITAL, BY

W. SAMS, ROYAL LIBRARY, ST. JAMES'S STREET.

MDCCCXXXIV.

Price Two Shillings and Sixpence, Stitched.

CHAPTER 18

Anatomy and Diseases of the Urinary and Sexual Organs *(1836)*

T he first edition of *Anatomy and Diseases of the Urinary and Sexual Organs* in 1836 comprised 284 pages and included three colour plates and five line drawings. As always in Guthrie's writings and lectures, many case histories added considerable interest to the text. The third and much smaller 1843 edition (Figure 18.1) had only two line drawings and was mainly concerned with the anatomy of the bladder and urethra, and the treatment of stricture. It 'endeavoured to render the directions for the treatment of each particular complaint so plain that anyone of even moderate capacity may understand and practise them'. It contained fewer case histories, was less verbose and was to be followed by a second part to include diseases of the prostate and the removal of stones from the bladder. The third edition will be described first.

1843 Edition

Chapter 1: Structure of the bladder

The following paragraph provides a flavour of Guthrie's less verbose style of writing (though typical of the time), but which nevertheless is interesting to read:

> The continual calls on the bladder in both sexes … under circumstances which are frequently foreign to their natural state, and the double function which the urethra has to perform in man, tend constantly to their derangement. The seeds of their decay are often caused to germinate at a much earlier period by the irregularities and vicious propensities of man himself. The diseases to which these parts are liable would be rarely experienced until the middle period of life was passed, if it were not for the indulgences and irregularities

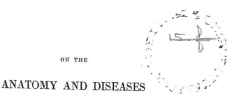

ON THE

ANATOMY AND DISEASES

OF THE

U R I N A R Y

AND

S E X U A L   O R G A N S.

BEING THE

FIRST PART OF THE LECTURES DELIVERED IN THE

Theatre of the Royal College of Surgeons

IN THE YEAR 1830;

AND

IN THE WESTMINSTER HOSPITAL IN 1833 & 1834.

BY

G. J. GUTHRIE, F. R. S.

Surgeon to the Westminster Hospital, and to the Royal Westminster Ophthalmic
Hospital, &c. &c. &c.

LONDON:
J. CHURCHILL, PRINCE'S STREET, SOHO.
1836.

Figure 18.1 *Title page of* Anatomy and Diseases of the Urinary and Sexual Organs, *published in 1843 (reproduced with permission from the Royal Society of Medicine, London)*

which usually prevail in a highly civilised community. They are always, when severe, the source of great anxiety of mind and distress of body ... and terminating not infrequently in a protracted and painful dissolution. Surgery can often afford great relief ... and is a source of no less satisfaction to the surgeon than of delight and of happiness to the patient. I know of no disease for the cure of which the gratitude of one man to another is more often and more cordially expressed.

This is followed by a basic description of the anatomy of the bladder and prostate.

Chapter 2: Structure of the urethra

Guthrie described a muscle previously incompletely described by anatomists – it was later known as 'Guthrie's muscle' – a *constrictor urethrae*, situated at the base of the bladder (fully described in *The Lancet*[1]). Guthrie showed by dissections that it was attached to the pubic and ischial ramus, that it completely surrounded the urethra and acted as a sphincter. This muscle had been described previously by Santorini but had almost ceased to be recognized.

Catheters and silver and gum-elastic bougies (Figure 18.2) are described, how they should be passed and the difficulties which may be encountered in introducing them.

Chapter 3: Formation of spasmodic and permanent stricture

Spasmodic strictures were often inflammatory in origin and could usually be dilated by a catheter. They might follow a bout of heavy drinking (a 'debauch') and could often be relieved by a hot bath. Guthrie had been called for advice by a Scottish friend

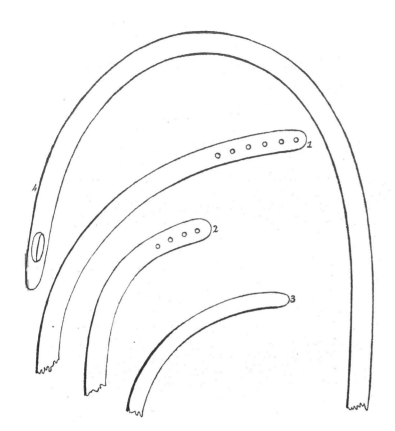

Figure 18.2 *(1 and 2) Prostate catheters; (3) solid sound; (4) elastic catheter and its stilet*

after such an episode and had advised this latter treatment. 'Damn you, Doctor, pass the catheter. I have had this treatment before', said his friend. Guthrie passed a catheter and drew off the water, upon which his friend jumped for joy saying, 'God bless you, Doctor, but damn the physic'. Permanent strictures required repeated dilatation.

Much of the substance of Chapter 3 was given in a lecture to the Medical Society of London and reported in *The Lancet*.[2]

Chapter 4: Symptoms and cure of a stricture

The symptoms of a stricture and its natural history are graphically described, reminiscent of his compassionate description of a hospital ward during the Peninsular War (see Chapter 2, p. 23). Repeated episodes of cystitis occur and later:

> The bladder cannot empty itself, it becomes distended behind the stricture, keeping the patient wet, uncomfortable, often excoriated – an object of disgust to all

around him. The straining which is necessary to expel the urine gives rise to a rupture and he is obliged to wear a truss. His miseries are only now beginning. The mucous membrane of the bowel protrudes and this, combined with bleeding piles, augments his distress. The cup of misery is not yet full. The desire to make water is continual. Worn down by his sufferings, in the agony of despair he prays to God for his dissolution and he seeks the temporary relief of laudanum. *[If a catheter is not passed the bladder may rupture and]* the urine is effused into the surrounding parts. ... The patient is sensible that his urine is flowing from his bladder ... but on looking down, he perceives with alarm that the scrotum and the neighbouring parts are greatly distended. He is for the time relieved, exciting hopes which are not likely to be realised. The white colour and doughy feel of the scrotum are succeeded by a dark red hue ... and must slough away with its covering skin ... and the patient often sinks and dies.

How to examine the urethra and what information might be obtained was also described. 'Model bougies, the point of which is made of softer material than the shaft', were used to define the exact position of the stricture so that a more rigid one, bent at an appropriate angle, could be passed to attempt dilatation (Figure 18.3).

The treatment of a stricture by dilatation or by caustics (argentum nitratum or potassa fusa) was discussed and Guthrie thought that there had been many prejudices against their use; the caustics were placed at the end of a bougie and applied to the stricture for one minute. These two caustics 'have fallen into obloquy and almost consequent disuse. Like most other prejudices they have some foundation in truth; but it is the *abuse* of caustics, and not the *use* of them which has given rise to this opinion'.

Many informative case histories were included, as in all of Guthrie's writings.

Chapter 5: Treatment of impassable stricture

Two different methods of treatment were advised. Guthrie wrote that 'long continued and equable pressure made on the face of the stricture by a pliable, hollow gum-elastic bougie, or by steady pressure made for a short time at intervals with a solid instrument until the obstruction is overcome' was required.

If the stricture could not be dilated Guthrie recommended and described in detail an operation through the perineum

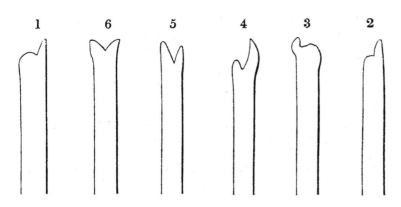

Figure 18.3 *(1–3) Impressions of the face of three different strictures, and these indicate the 'remains of the natural passages by the prominent points in each'. (4–6) Show the 'remains of the natural passage and the commencement of a false passage in each, the edge of the stricture causing the hollow between the prominences'*

which had been introduced by Astley Cooper into surgical practice and had been first carried out in 1793: 'It can usually be done in 3–4 minutes'. A sound was passed into the urethra and 'held steadily against the stricture'. With the left forefinger inserted into the rectum the perineum was opened anterior to the rectum, the urethra was exposed and incised between the prostate and the stricture, which was also divided. An indwelling catheter was left in place.

If a bougie could be passed through the stricture an attempt might be made to cut it with a special knife attached to the end of a sound.

Chapter 6: Suppression and retention of urine

A discussion of suppression (anuria) and retention of urine was followed by the treatment of the latter by catheterization, or by operation if this failed. The choice of treatment was discussed. The sequence of events following urinary retention was graphically described:

> The urine may drop from the urethra, the bed clothes may be wet from it ... the kidneys secrete more than is discharged and are willing to secrete still more if the pressure on them which prevents it is taken off. The bladder is distending and the rupture of the urethra is at hand. The agony which the patient endures is great, the anxiety of countenance is strongly marked, the general distress and the great sympathy of the whole system are too fearfully expressed to be mistaken. The bladder may be felt rising high above the pubes and descending into the rectum ... and the surgeon has only the choice of his operation left.

Five operations to alleviate this situation had been recommended by different authors:

> 1st to puncture the bladder above the pubes; 2nd to puncture through the rectum; 3rd to open the urethra from without; 4th to divide the stricture and re-establish the passage by an instrument passed along the urethra; or 5th by a judicious combination of both these last methods.

Suprapubic puncture was considered by Guthrie to be dangerous, puncture through the rectum was 'easily performed' and its technique was described, using a curved trocar and cannula. However, Guthrie's preferred treatment was to apply 'gentle but steady pressure on the stricture with a catheter' and, if this failed, to open the urethra through the perineal approach described above in his fifth chapter: 'If the surgeon is unhappily too late and the urethra has given way by ulceration behind the stricture', the resulting situation is discussed; a 'fair and free incision must be made in the perineum until the superficial fascia is freely divided' to allow drainage.

Chapter 7: Irritation of the membranous and prostatic parts of the urethra

This chapter is mainly devoted to case histories and the cause and treatment of urethritis.

1836 Edition

Lecture 1: Structure of bladder.

Lecture 2: Structure of prostate – it is interesting to note that Guthrie said that a description of a new so-called middle lobe of the prostate by Sir Everard Home had already been described by John Hunter several years previously, antedating the now well-documented plagiarism of Hunter by Home (Figure 18.4).

Lectures 3–7: Strictures of the urethra and the passage of sounds through them (60 pages).

Lectures 8–12: Strictures of the membranous part of the urethra and their treatment (100 pages).

Lecture 13: Prostatic part of urethra.

Figure 18.4 *The so-called middle lobe (1) is thought by Guthrie to be really part of the left lateral lobe (2)*

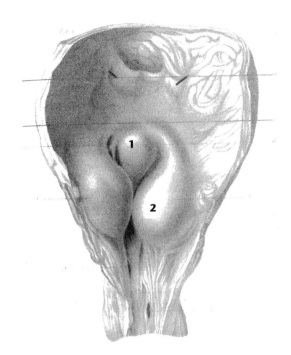

Lecture 14: Chronic enlargement of the prostate (Figure 18.5).

Lectures 15–16: Chronic thickening of neck of bladder – not now thought, as had been thought previously, to be due to middle lobe enlargement, and lucidly described by Guthrie:

> It may commence at an early period of life. It slumbers on like a smothered fire, ready at some future time to burst forth with renewed vigour and to lead to his destruction by the production of disease in the neighbouring parts.

References

1. *Lancet* 1833–4; **1**: 159, 163.
2. *Lancet* 1851; **1**: 477–9.

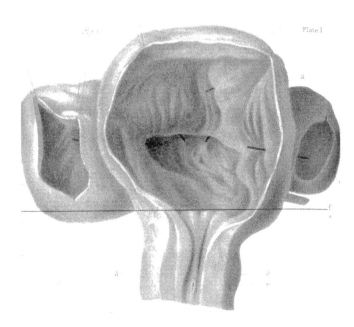

Figure 18.5 *Bladder with a diverticulum on each side*

CHAPTER 19

Compound Fractures of the Extremities *(1838)*

*C*ompound Fractures of the Extremities, a series of lectures delivered at the Westminster Hospital during 1836–8, was published in 1838 (Figure 19.1). It is a fascinating book of 64 pages, not so much because of its surgical content, which, though important, is remarkably little considering its title, but rather because of its absorbing personal record of events during Guthrie's service in the Peninsular War, his continued criticisms of the army medical service and its administration, personal recollections of patients he had previously treated, where to site regimental, brigade and general hospitals, and, on pages 24–5, the two episodes of his knowledge of navigation described in Chapter 1. The book provides a vivid insight into the conduct of warfare in the early 19th century, the privations endured by soldiers of all ranks, how battles were fought and the life and behaviour of the troops before and after each conflict. It also describes how the members of the medical service responded to battle situations, or were unable to respond because of poor administration and inefficiency of the army directorate.

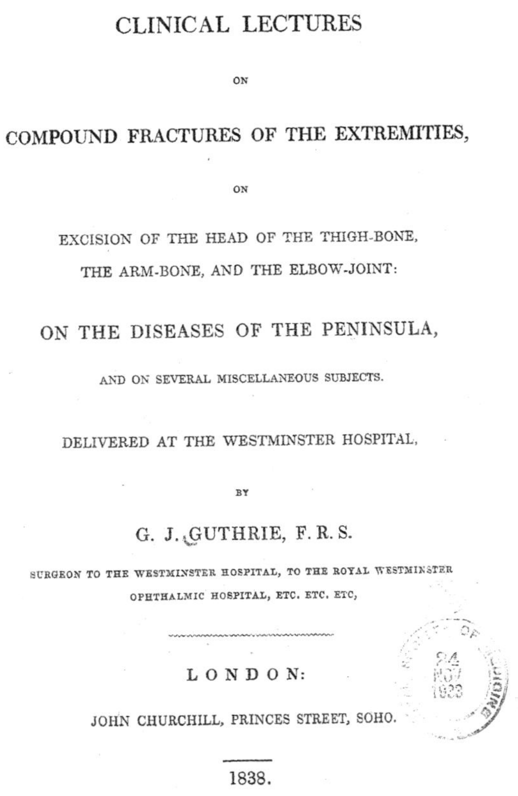

CLINICAL LECTURES

ON

COMPOUND FRACTURES OF THE EXTREMITIES,

ON

EXCISION OF THE HEAD OF THE THIGH-BONE,
THE ARM-BONE, AND THE ELBOW-JOINT:

ON THE DISEASES OF THE PENINSULA,

AND ON SEVERAL MISCELLANEOUS SUBJECTS.

DELIVERED AT THE WESTMINSTER HOSPITAL,

BY

G. J. GUTHRIE, F. R. S.

SURGEON TO THE WESTMINSTER HOSPITAL, TO THE ROYAL WESTMINSTER
OPHTHALMIC HOSPITAL, ETC. ETC. ETC,

LONDON:

JOHN CHURCHILL, PRINCES STREET, SOHO.

1838.

Figure 19.1 *Title page of* Compound Fractures of the Extremities, *published in 1838 (reproduced with permission from the Royal Society of Medicine, London)*

These lectures had been given free of charge for 22 years to members of the public services. In the Preface Guthrie empha- sizes that both he *and those attending the lectures* should be paid, as was done in Edinburgh and every other capital in Europe. If veterinary surgeons are paid for demonstrating 'how to cure the Horses of the Army, surely something of the same should be done for the Men'. There are no illustrations. The sixth lecture is almost entirely devoted to Guthrie's personal reminiscences of the Peninsular campaign, extracts of which are given in Chapter 3.

First clinical lecture

Sir Astley Cooper observed to me the other day that the last war had given the greatest impulse to surgery it had ever received in this country. Those who remained at home were obliged to labour and increase their knowledge that they might be enabled to teach; and those who went abroad were obliged to learn because they could not help it.

Guthrie then emphasizes four points in his surgical technique for amputation:

1. He preferred not to use a tourniquet but to rely on pressure on the main artery by an assistant.
2. The skin and fascia should be divided by an initial circular incision down to the muscles, so that painful dissection of the former is avoided.
3. The bone should be cut short – 'woe there is to the man to the end of whose bone the cicatrix adheres, he is unhappy for the rest of his life; he will not forget the doctor'.
4. The bone should be sawn perpendicularly to prevent its splintering.

This occupies one page only of the five-page Introductory Lecture – the remainder describes various episodes during the Peninsular War.

Second clinical lecture: Peculiar and unde- scribed injury of the shoulder

This injury was described as a fracture of the head of the humerus caused by a fall on the elbow, pushing the head of the humerus into its socket in the scapula, and was not associated with much limitation of movement.

Third clinical lecture: Compound fractures and gunshot fractures of the arm

How to examine the injury is described, followed by an emphasis on the removal of splintered pieces of bone to prevent later sequestrum formation. It is also emphasized that amputation is not required for many of these cases, as had been formerly advised, providing the blood supply to the arm is not compromised; if the head of the humerus or the elbow joint only had been fractured, it should be excised. After elbow joint excision the forearm should be 'brought into the bent position'. In both cases the patient would then have a useful arm.

Fourth clinical lecture: Compound and gunshot fractures of the thigh

Amputation, though often necessary in these cases, is 'an opprobrium of surgery'. Of 43 fractured thighs after the battle of Toulouse only 18 retained their limbs and three months later only five had useful limbs; many would have preferred to have had an amputation. The importance of primary (immediate) amputation is emphasized, as also that of the use of a straight, rather than the customary bent, splint.

Fifth clinical lecture: Excision of the head of the thigh bone

Precise instructions for excision of the head of the femur are given, an operation which in many cases would avoid amputation. Guthrie had not done this operation himself 'in a living man', but he was convinced that in the future it should be done following a gunshot wound of this joint.

Sixth clinical lecture: Excision of the elbow joint

This lecture is the shortest in the book and only one of its five pages is devoted to excision of the elbow joint. The remainder is part of Guthrie's account of the Peninsular War and includes an interesting case of haemoptysis due to an inhaled leech, a soldier who nearly died after accidentally swallowing a living salamander, an episode in which he was nearly killed because of mistaken identity, and finally a dinner in a monastery, during which one of the monks was seduced by an English lady (see Chapter 3).

A shortened account of Guthrie's very precise and clear instructions for this excision of the elbow joint is worthy of inclusion:

The cases which require this operation are those in which the articulating ends of the humerus, radius and ulna are wholly or in part so much injured that little or no hope remains of a successful result. These cases have usually been submitted to amputation on account of serious injuries to joints being rarely cured. The object of excision is to save the forearm, and the situation of the shot-hole or holes does not signify much as to the manner of operating. The principal point regulating the proceeding is to preserve the nerves entire; and the most important one likely to be injured is the ulnar.

To avoid this, which lies between the olecranon and the internal condyle ... a common straight but strong pointed knife is to be pushed into the joint, immediately above and close to the olecranon process ... the incision thus begun is to be carried outwardly to the external part of the humerus, dividing thereby the tendinous insertion of the triceps. From the end of this transverse incision a cut is to be made perpendicularly upwards and downwards, about an inch and a half each way, and the same is to be done at the other end of the of the transverse cut. The whole will now resemble the letter H and the two flaps thus formed must be turned up and down. The olecranon may now be readily sawn off. Before this is done the ulnar nerve must be carefully separated from its attachments and turned aside that it may not be injured. This exposes the joint effectively, and the head of the radius may now be cut through by the saw, or large scissors in the case of old standing disease, and separated from the lateral ligament and the humerus, care being taken not to cut, if possible, the insertion of the biceps into its tubercle. The articulating extremity of the humerus ought now to be pushed through the wound and the broken end sawn off or removed, so as to leave it quite smooth. The brachial artery and median nerve are out of all reasonable distance for injury, and to prevent the possibility of its occurrence a knife or a spatula may be placed underneath, close to the bone and quite across, before the saw is applied.

The articulating cartilaginous broken ends of the bones having been thus removed ... the forearm is to be bent and the ends of the radius and ulna are to be brought into apposition with the extremity of the humerus. The incisions are to be brought together by stitches and sticking plaster, duly supported by compress and bandage. Mr Syme strongly advises that strict attention should be paid to procure union of the transverse incision just above the olecranon; for a broad cicatrix interferes with the motion of the joint, a reasonable degree of which is always to be expected in a successful case. The arm should be duly supported by a proper sling. As the shot-holes must remain open any discharge of blood or serum which takes place will readily pass through them.

Passive motion should be early given to the parts so as to favour the formation of a false joint, but this should be carefully and moderately done. A fixed or stiff joint is not to be desired but if it cannot be avoided it must be procured with the forearm at a right angle with the arm when it will be most serviceable. The patient is best placed on his face on a bed or a table, which renders the steps of the operation more convenient to the operator.

Seventh clinical lecture: Diseases of the Peninsula to which the British troops were exposed in 1811 and 1812

This is a long lecture concerned with heat exhaustion, general hygiene, the importance of adequate nutrition, the logistics of troop movement and the avoidance of irregular pay, so that when received it is not all spent on alcohol for several days with the inevitable consequences.

CHAPTER 20

Injuries of the Head Affecting the Brain and The Anatomy and Surgery of Inguinal and Femoral Hernia *(1847)*

*I*njuries of the Head Affecting the Brain and The Anatomy and Surgery of Inguinal and Femoral Hernia were published together in one volume in 1847 by John Churchill (Figure 20.1). Five years previously *Injuries of the Head Affecting the Brain* had been published alone. The books recorded lectures given at the Royal College of Surgeons in 1831 and 1841.

Injuries of the Head Affecting the Brain

The text of this section comprised 155 pages (8 × 11 inches – large by 19th century custom for medical books) summarizing Guthrie's lectures to the Royal College of Surgeons in 1841. The contents included general remarks, definition of concussion and compression of the brain, simple fractures, fractures of the base of the skull and inner table, wounds of the scalp, depressed

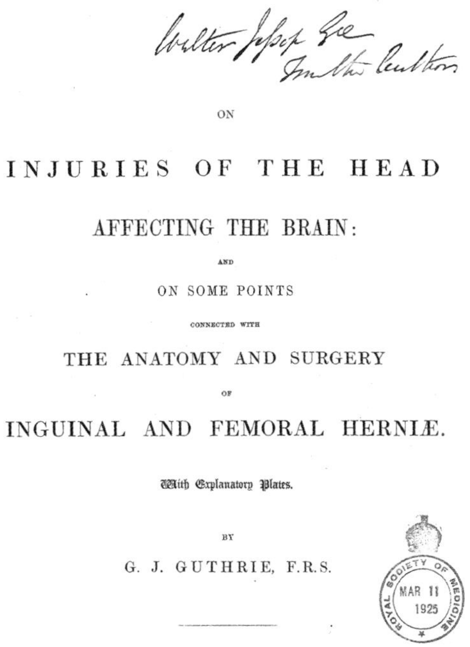

Figure 20.1 *Title page of* Injuries of the Head Affecting the Brain and The Anatomy and Surgery of Inguinal and Femoral Hernia, *published in 1847 (reproduced with permission from the Royal Society of Medicine)*

ON

INJURIES OF THE HEAD

AFFECTING THE BRAIN:

AND

ON SOME POINTS

CONNECTED WITH

THE ANATOMY AND SURGERY

OF

INGUINAL AND FEMORAL HERNIÆ.

With Explanatory Plates.

BY

G. J. GUTHRIE, F.R.S.

LONDON:
JOHN CHURCHILL, PRINCES STREET, SOHO;
AND
HENRY RENSHAW, 356, STRAND.
M DCCC XLVII.
Price Seven Shillings, boards.

fractures of the skull, contre-coup injuries of the brain, gunshot wounds of the skull, and protrusion (fungus) of the brain following penetrating wounds. The text was one continuous narrative, with no chapter headings and few paragraphs, and this made for very tedious reading.

A preliminary statement that 'injuries of the head affecting the brain are difficult of distinction, doubtful in their character, treacherous in their course and for the most part fatal in their results' was followed by a description of patients treated by Guthrie and other English and European surgeons, some of whom had made a surprising and remarkable recovery. The comments on treatment were somewhat superficial but this was understandable considering the state of knowledge of brain injury in the early 19th century, much of which had stemmed from the work of Le Dran and Petit in the previous century in France, with a further contribution from Abernethy later in England.

Middle meningeal haemorrhage was described, together with its successful treatment by trepanation (elevation of a portion of bone) or by trephination (removal of a disc of bone), during which damage to the underlying dura was less likely.

Numerous case histories were described and it was apparent that Guthrie must have had an extensive knowledge of the treatment of head injuries. He emphasized two aspects of head injury: (1) a fracture of the vertex of the skull was less serious than a fracture of the base of the skull; and (2) frontal skull injuries were more dangerous than lateral injuries, and both were less dangerous than posterior injuries.

A remarkable head injury with recovery in 1403

The head injury of the 16-year-old Prince Henry (the future Henry V) at the battle of Shrewsbury in 1403 has been recorded elsewhere,[1,2] but it is worthy of inclusion here because the injury is not well known and because of the ingenious operation which was carried out which led to his remarkable recovery. The Prince had sustained an arrow injury to the left of his nose, the shaft had been removed but the arrow head had remained six inches deep 'in the bone at the back of the skull'. John Bradmore, the King's surgeon, had been consulted and, by devising a small pair of hollow tongs which incorporated a screw mechanism, he had managed to extract it: 'then, by moving it to and fro, little by little (with the help of God), I extracted the arrowhead'. The wound healed after 20 days (so it is related! But the Prince survived and the arrow must have entered his upper jaw, *not* his skull). Nevertheless it was a remarkable operation in the 15th century. The Prince was very lucky.

The Anatomy and Surgery of Inguinal and Femoral Hernia

This second section comprised 37 pages and three plates (each of which had a detailed description) and summarized Guthrie's lectures at the Royal College of Surgeons in 1831 on the anatomy of this region. Again, the text of this section was one continuous narrative. The anatomical dissections had been made by Owen and Astley Cooper, and the plates had been drawn by William Clift, John Hunter's assistant. A detailed description of each plate was included.

The descriptions of the anatomy of the inguinal canal by Astley Cooper, Lawrence, Scarpa, Hesselbach, Cloquet, Velpau and Langenbeck had all differed and Guthrie thought that 'the reader cannot fail to be surprised at the great difference which exists between these different versions of the same thing'. Students of anatomy would have concluded that 'the descriptions are not sufficiently clear and distinct, if not in some cases faulty', or even that no one description could have fitted all cases, for the anatomy might have been very variable. An extensive discussion of these descriptions, especially that of the *fascia transversalis* (first described by Astley Cooper), was followed by Guthrie's own opinion of the anatomy of this region, which he illustrated (Figures 20.2 and 20.3).

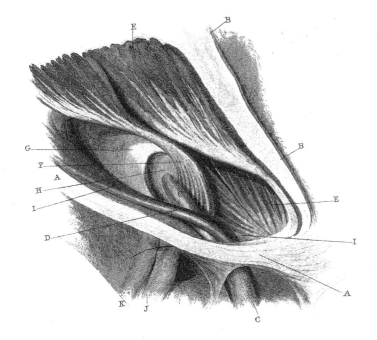

Figure 20.2 *Anatomy of inguinal hernia (drawn by William Clift, John Hunter's assistant, after a dissection made by Sir Astley Cooper) (Figure 1, Plate 2 in the book). A, Poupart's ligament; B, tendon of external oblique muscle; C, spermatic cord; D, cremaster muscle; E, internal oblique muscle; F, transversalis muscle; G, fascia transversalis; H, peritoneum; I, inferior fibres of transversalis muscle; J and K, femoral vein and artery*

Figure 20.3 *Anatomy of inguinal hernia as described by Sir Astley Cooper (Figure 3 in book, drawn by William Clift, John Hunter's assistant). A, Poupart's ligament; B, internal oblique muscle; C, transversalis muscle; D, cremaster muscle; E, rectus muscle; H, spermatic cord; I, internal ring; K, external ring*

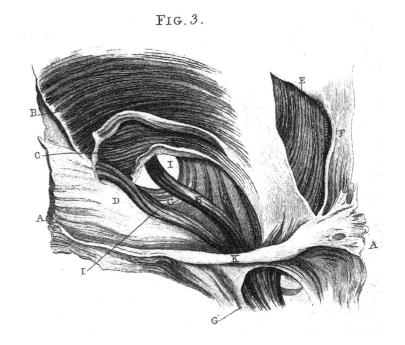

FIG. 3.

The treatment of a strangulated hernia was discussed, the object being to relax the contraction of the transversalis muscle around the inner ring by a combination of venesection, a warm bath and a tobacco enema. Failure of this treatment required division of the inner ring of the transversalis muscle and Guthrie described his preferred technique for this operation.

References

1. Barker J. *Agincourt.* London: Little, Brown, 2005, p. 29.
2. Beck RT. *The Cutting Edge: Early History of the Surgeons of London.* London: Lund Humphries, 1974, pp. 13, 75–6, 117.

CHAPTER 21

Wounds and Injuries of the Abdomen and the Pelvis
(1847)

ounds and Injuries of the Abdomen and the Pelvis (Figure 21.1) was published in 1847 and later in articles in *The Lancet.*[1] There are 73 pages of rather small print and there are no illustrations. There are 113 case reports of these injuries, most of which Guthrie had treated, though also included are many cases treated by Astley Cooper and John Bell in England and Scotland, by Larrey, Percy, Petit, Dupuytren and Le Dran in Paris, Langenbech and Schmidt in Berlin and several from America.

In the Preface Guthrie says that he had suffered 'the greatest calamity which could possibly have befallen' him (his wife had died from cholera the previous year) and that in writing these case histories he 'had drawn some consolation by beguiling away my winter evenings in preparing them for the press, with the hope and belief that they may be useful, not only by pointing out what has been done to the present time, but by drawing attention to what ought perhaps hereafter to be done under similar circumstances'.

The variety of injuries makes fascinating reading and includes musket ball and sabre wounds, and impalement and self-inflicted wounds – some of the patients made a remarkable and complete recovery. In many cases the aftercare is also described and this

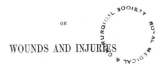

ON

WOUNDS AND INJURIES

OF THE

ABDOMEN AND THE PELVIS;

BEING THE

SECOND PART

OF THE

LECTURES ON SOME OF THE MORE IMPORTANT POINTS
IN SURGERY.

By G. J. GUTHRIE, F.R.S.

LONDON:
J. CHURCHILL, PRINCES STREET, SOHO.
HENRY RENSHAW, 356, STRAND.
1847.
[PRICE THREE SHILLINGS.]

Figure 21.1 *Title page of* Wounds and Injuries of the Abdomen and the Pelvis, *published in 1847 (reproduced with permission from the Royal Society of Medicine, London)*

contributes an interesting commentary on the medical treatment at that time, as does the background to some of the injuries. Guthrie's comments on the treatment of many cases are included, some critical and some not.

Especially interesting are case 3 (drainage of a psoas abscess into bladder), case 13 (abdominal transfixion injury), cases 21 and 22 (protrusion of bowel after abdominal injury, following which patient walked to doctor), case 25 (thoraco-abdominal wound in a child), cases 31 and 32 (self-inflicted injury to abdominal wall, with protrusion of bowel), case 39 (officer wounded in abdomen, who rode to hospital 'with his bowel wrapped in his shirt'), cases 50–52 (musket ball injury to abdomen, and ball later passed *per anum*), case 62 (knife wound of stomach), and cases 81 and 82 (kidney wound with external urinary fistula).

Dr J. Hennen Snr (1779–1828), who treated several of these injuries, was an army surgeon in the Peninsular War and at Waterloo. He published *Observations on the Practice of Military Surgery* in 1818 and died from yellow fever in Gibraltar in 1828 with the rank of Deputy Inspector. He assisted Guthrie at the first successful amputation of the hip joint after the battle of Waterloo.

Guthrie's 'general conclusions' for the treatment of these injuries were:

1. Severe blows may lead to ventral hernia.
2. Abdominal wall abscesses should be opened as early as possible to prevent infection spreading into the peritoneal cavity.
3. The liver and spleen are very liable to rupture following a severe blow.
4. Incised wounds frequently cause a ventral hernia.
5. Lacerations of abdominal wall muscle should be repaired by a continuous suture through the integument only, not through the muscle.
6. Sutures should never be inserted through the whole abdominal wall.
7. Purgatives should not be given after a penetrating wound of the abdomen; enemata are to be preferred.
8. Protruded omentum should always be returned to the abdomen and not be excised.
9. A punctured intestine requires no immediate treatment, but if more than a third of its circumference has been damaged it should be closed with a continuous suture.

10. The patient should be inclined towards the injured side.

11. 'If the belly swells' the sutures should be cut to allow 'the offending matter to be released'.

12. If the incised wound is small and there is considerable effusion within the abdomen the wound should be enlarged.

13. Retained musket balls should be 'sought for and removed, if it can be done with propriety and safety'.

14. If the bladder is injured an indwelling gum-elastic catheter is necessary.

15. If a catheter cannot be passed an opening in the perineum should be made to allow escape of urine (see also Chapter 18, p. 236).

16. All abdominal injuries should be treated by the greatest possible abstinence from food, and in some cases from drink, and the frequent administration of enemata.

Lecture 1

Cases 1 and 2: Severe blunt injury to abdomen, followed several months later by a ventral hernia.

Case 3: Psoas abscess which eventually drained into the bladder.

Case 4: Severe infected wound of anterior abdominal wall, but spread of infection into abdomen prevented by resistance of peritoneum.

Case 5: Sabre wound of anterior abdominal wall near ensiform cartilage, which penetrated stomach. Patient recovered. Small persisting hernia at site of injury.

Case 6: Horse caught his foot in a rabbit hole and soldier thrown over horse's head. Soldier died. Post-mortem showed ruptured liver and large haemoperitoneum.

Case 7: Kick from a horse above pubis, leading to abdominal distension. Patient died 24 hours later. Post-mortem showed laceration of ileum. Purgatives had increased the distension and are therefore contraindicated.

Cases 8 and 9: Blunt injury to abdominal wall in two children. Distension followed and both died. Post-mortem showed laceration of small intestine. 'The tympanitic state of the abdomen in these two cases is considered pathognomonic of laceration of the small intestine'.

Case 10: Patient knocked down by a carriage, one wheel of which ran over abdomen. Abdomen became distended, patient 'bled and leeched several times'. Patient died two months later. Post-mortem showed ruptured small intestine.

Case 11: Cannon shot to right side of abdomen leading to severe bruising. Patient died 12 hours later. Post-mortem showed ruptured right kidney and haemoperitoneum.

Case 12: Blunt injury to abdominal wall leading to severe abdominal distension. Patient died two weeks later. Post-mortem showed laceration of intestine.

Case 13: Transfixion injury by a ramrod; entry two inches below umbilicus and exit wound posteriorly after penetrating second lumbar vertebra. Rod extracted. Patient recovered. Two other civilian transfixion injuries treated by other authors are reported; both recovered.

Cases 14–16: Protrusion of omentum following penetrating abdominal wound. Omentum returned to abdomen. Patients recovered.

Case 17: Musket ball injury to abdomen. Entry and exit wounds on opposite sides. Ball carried with it part of omentum. Protruded omentum gradually receded spontaneously into abdomen. Patient recovered. Discussion of treatment of protruded omentum.

Case 18: Knife wound to abdomen resulting in protrusion of small intestine. Replaced into abdomen. Patient recovered.

Case 19 (of Dr Long, Arthurstown, Ireland): Large knife wound in abdomen leading to protrusion of omentum, stomach and colon. Replaced back into abdomen. Patient recovered.

Case 20 (of Dr Worthington, USA): Two wounds to abdomen, one eight inches long above inguinal ligament and another smaller one below umbilicus. Eighteen inches of colon and 30 inches of small intestine protruded through the larger wound and 'a small fold of intestine' protruded through the smaller wound. Intestine replaced. Patient recovered.

Case 21 (of Rosier de Landon): Boy gored by horn of a bull, causing a wound from groin to umbilicus through which intestine protruded. Replaced. 'Next morning the boy walked three miles to see the doctor, carrying the bowel which had again protruded in his shirt'. Bowel replaced. Patient recovered in three weeks.

Case 22 (of Madame Doucat) (in early 18th century): Soldier had been struck by a battleaxe in abdomen 'through which a great part of his bowels protruded and which he carried in his hat enveloped in his shirt'. Walked 3–4 miles to see Madame Doucat. Intestine replaced and wound sewn up with a 'well waxed silken thread'. Patient recovered.

Cases 23 and 24: Small sword wounds to abdominal wall; small intestine protruded and was replaced. Patients recovered.

Guthrie concludes that:

> Wounds of the cavity of the abdomen require the strictest care, an unremitting attention, and yet occasionally baffle all skill and knowledge; whilst at others they appear to set all rules and all received opinions at defiance.

Lecture 2

This lecture is preceded by a discussion of early attempts at intestinal anastomosis.

Case 25 (of Mr Calton, Newark, Scotland): Thoraco-abdominal wound caused by a boar tusk in a child aged seven. Stomach, omentum and much of the intestine protruded. The 'ileum was torn across'. Ileum repaired with four sutures. Patient recovered. [A remarkable case.]
  Other similar cases from England and France are described and discussed.

Case 26 (of Prof. Cloquet and others): Cases of repair of accidental injury to intestine whilst operating on a strangulated hernia.

Case 27 (of M. Baudens): Musket ball injury to abdomen; separate entry and exit wounds. Large hole seen in colon when patient made to cough. Repair. Patient recovered.
  Discussion of similar cases seen by other surgeons.

Cases 28–30 (of Nancianti, Naples): Cases of strangulated hernia in which intestine had been torn during attempt at reduction or during operation. Intestine repaired. Patient recovered.

Two self-inflicted injuries to abdominal wall

Case 31: Injury with a pair of scissors to abdominal wall and 17 inches of intestine cut off. At operation intestine returned to abdomen without any hope of recovery. But she did recover! Died six months later 'without any symptoms of disease'. ? Why. Post-mortem showed that part of the colon had been cut off and the ends had become united by a small passage large enough to permit passage of semi-liquid faeces.

Case 32: Attempted suicide by razor cut to abdomen and two and a half inches of colon were seen to be lying on the floor. Ends of colon joined together with a continuous suture. Abdominal wound closed. Transferred by hand barrow from 'his wretched garret without anyone to look after him' to hospital, a distance of over one mile. Patient recovered.

Lecture 3

This lecture is preceded by further discussion on intestinal injuries.

Case 33: Sabre wound to abdominal wall; repaired and patient recovered.

Case 34: Severe thoraco-abdominal wound. Patient died soon after admission.

Case 35: (of Dr Sharmen, Rotherham). Penknife wound of abdomen six inches long. Large quantity of intestine protruded. Bowel returned. Patient recovered.

> The following cases (cases 36–52) of the survivors of the hundreds who died under similar circumstances between 1808 (battle of Roliça) and Waterloo (1815) may be read with a melancholy interest as showing what may happen in a few rare instances; and even then as more dependant on the wantonness of nature than on the united efforts of science and art.

Cases 36–48: Separate entry and exit wounds, the ball having 'traversed the body'.

Case 36: 'In a soldier of the brigade of heavy cavalry under General Le Marchant advancing in line to charge the French cavalry at Salamanca (on which occasion the General was killed)'. Musket ball injury; entry near umbilicus and exit posteriorly having traversed the abdomen. Protruded intestine replaced. Patient recovered.

Case 37 (of Dr Hennen): Grapeshot injury across anterior part of abdomen 'without injury to the bowel, a portion of which protruded at each opening'. Wound healed slowly. Patient recovered.

Case 38: Small musket ball injury, entry below umbilicus, exit near spine. Patient recovered.

Case 39: Pistol ball injury. Entry at left hip and exit below umbilicus on right. He dismounted from his horse and found 'there was a protrusion of bowel from wound in front and copious haemorrhage from the wound in the back'. He had to remount his horse quickly as a French officer called out, 'Rendez-vous, mon officier', to which he replied, 'Pas encore, Monsieur', and quickly rode away. He was compelled to wrap the protrusion into his shirt and keep it in as much as he could with one hand. At the field hospital the protrusion was returned to the abdomen. A few weeks later he and a few other wounded were evacuated 'in bullock carts, and a desperate journey it was'. After prolonged sick leave in England he rejoined his regiment at Waterloo. [Included in this report is a long and vivid account by Lt Slater-Smith of his injury and convalescence.]

Case 40: Musket ball injury; entry above umbilicus and exit close to lumbar vertebra. During next few days he developed what would now be recognized as a paralytic ileus, which subsided after 10 days. Patient recovered.

Cases 41–43: Musket ball injuries to anterior abdomen. External faecal fistulae developed and these subsequently closed. Patients recovered.

Case 44 (of Baron Larrey): Musket ball injury to abdominal wall. Intestine protruded and became strangulated; this was relieved with scissors. Patient recovered.

Cases 45 and 46: Musket ball injuries; entry and exit wounds on opposite sides of anterior abdominal wall. Faecal fistulae gradually closed. Patients recovered.

Dr Thomson (a Peninsular War and Waterloo surgeon) summarized his views on this type of injury after Waterloo: 'the more that is left to nature in the progress of reunion and the less her operations are interfered with, the greater will be the chance of ultimate recovery'. Guthrie added that this is correct providing there are no clear indications for interference, but when they are present 'the do-nothing system is generally followed by death'.

Case 47: Gunshot wound to abdomen – entry and exit wounds below umbilicus. Patient died next day. No post-mortem.

Case 48: Abdominal wound. Entry and exit wounds below umbilicus. Intestine protruded from both wounds, was replaced and wound was dressed. Faecal fistula six days later 'and patient sank and died'. No post-mortem.

Case 49 (of La Motte): Penetrating epigastric wound by shot. Simple dressing to wound. Symptoms of peritonitis five days later and patient died. Post-mortem showed three minute wounds of ileum.

Cases 50–52: Three cases of musket ball passed later via anus.

Case 50: Musket ball injury with entry wound posteriorly near iliac crest, followed by faecal fistula which slowly closed. On fifth day ball passed *per anum* and later, on several occasions, pieces of his coat and breeches. Patient recovered.

Case 51: Musket ball injury below and to right of umbilicus. Ten days later ball 'passed with faeces'. Wound healed after three weeks. Eventual recovery.

Case 52: Musket ball injury at Waterloo just below umbilicus. Walked to a nearby village and passed ball six days later *per anum*. Then marched with his regiment to Paris. Several weeks later felt something blocking his anus and found it was part of the waistband of his breeches. Patient recovered.

Lecture 4

Case 53 (of M. Cabrol, Montpellier): Self-inflicted injury to liver in 1604, causing severe haemorrhage. Infected haemoperitoneum later. Drained. Patient recovered.

Case 54 (reported by Petit, Paris): Sword injury below xiphoid. Fever 12 days later due to swelling below wound. Incised and one and a half pints of blood released. Patient recovered.

Cases 55–57 (of M. Ravaton, France): Three cases of localized peritonitis and abscess formation following penetrating sword wounds. Drained. Patients recovered.

Case 58 (of Dr Stuart): Sword wound resulting in death from peritonitis seven days later. Post-mortem showed sword had penetrated gall bladder.

Case 59 (of Sabatier, Paris): Similar to case 58.

Case 60 (of M. Biot, France): Intra-abdominal abscess between iliac crest and umbilicus. Incised and drained. Several days later two large *lumbrici* (worms) came out of wound, following which a faecal fistula developed. Then a suprapubic abscess which was drained. Another faecal fistula developed. After 57 days fistulae and wounds all closed and 'natural passage [of faeces] was restored'.

Case 61 (of Mr Fryer, Stamford): Violent blow in region of liver, followed four days later by jaundice. Three weeks after injury abdomen became very distended. Trocar and cannula inserted and 13 pints of bile removed, 12 days later 15 pints, 9 days later 13 pints and 18 days later 6 pints, after which gradual recovery occurred.

Case 62 (of Dr Archer, Maryland, USA): Knife wound penetrating stomach, from which 'his dinner discharged through the incision'. External wound closed. Nine days later abscess in groin incised and cabbage evacuated. Patient recovered.

Case 63 (of Dr Fuschtires, England): Acute pain in abdomen and a hard mass felt in right hypochondrium. Laparotomy revealed an intussusception. Intestine was unfolded 'to the extent of two feet'. Intestinal wound closed. Patient recovered.

Case 64 (of Dr Manlove, Boston): Intestinal obstruction by a band, relieved by laparotomy.

Case 65 (of Dr Maclean): Operation to relieve strangulated hernia. Four days after operation wound opened up when patient strained at stool and intestine protruded. Intestine returned to abdominal cavity but faecal fistula developed. This eventually closed and patient recovered.

Case 66 (of Mr Hilton, Essex): Intestinal obstruction in a young man. Previous history of peritonitis. Obstruction partially relieved by 'metallic mercury'. At laparotomy in patient's home six inches of small intestine had become strangulated by a band. Obstruction relieved. Patient died nine hours after operation, which had lasted one hour. [This operation was performed in 1846; ether was first used in 1842. ? Anaesthesia for this procedure.]
    Similar cases reported by Larrey, Baudens and other surgeons in France are described.

Case 67: Strangulated ileum by a band. No operation. Post-mortem findings described. The opinions of Larrey and Baudens on this type of case are included.

Lecture 5

These case reports are preceded by a discussion of the necessity for a colostomy after abdominal wounds or strangulated hernia operations. There was little experience of this in England but much in France.

Case 68 (of M. Huttier, France): Musket ball injury to abdomen two years previously – complete recovery. Patient died from pneumonia. Post-mortem showed ball in gall bladder, which showed no sign of injury.

Case 69 (of M. Poroisse, France): Two sabre wounds to upper abdomen after a duel, followed by profuse haemorrhage, and patient appeared to be dying. Very large haematoma evacuated and 'respiration and circulation appeared to be relieved'. Patient recovered after three weeks.

Case 70: Musket ball wound causing liver injury and fractured lower ribs. Five years after injury several attacks of acute abdominal pain when patient bent forward, relieved by a metal brace to prevent this movement.

Case 71 (of Dr Hennen): Musket ball injury to right chest – posterior entry wound (with fracture of eighth and ninth ribs) and anterior exit wound. Evidence of lung injury as patient expectorated sputum tinged with bile. Slow improvement began after repeated venesection over a period of five weeks. Complete recovery after two months.

Cases 72–77: Injury to liver.

Case 72 (of Dr Blicke): Musket ball injury to right eighth rib causing liver injury. 'Bilious discharge' and haemorrhage for two months from wound, which completely healed two weeks later. Treatment by venesection.

Case 73 (of Mr Bruce): Musket ball injury to upper abdomen, causing liver damage, as shown by discharge of bile from wound. This gradually ceased over two months. Retained ball never found.

Case 74 (of Mr Ryan): Musket ball injury with entry wound over liver and posterior exit wound. Repeated venesection. One month later both wounds healed.

Case 75: Musket ball injury with entry wound over liver and posterior exit wound. 'Considered hopeless'. Copious blood and bile discharge. Repeated venesection. Gradual improvement over following weeks. Patient recovered.

Case 76: Musket ball wound to liver; copious blood and bile discharge. 'Given up as lost'. But gradual improvement occurred. Patient returned to England and seen annually for several years. Continued discharge of pus and bile from wound, together with frequent attacks of pain. Ball in liver could be felt with a probe and Guthrie hoped it would be discharged. He considered trying to remove it with a long pair of forceps. Patient failed one of his usual appointments and 'probably died during one of his attacks of pain'.

Case 77 (of Dr Roux, France): Knife wound to upper abdomen and a cut two inches long could be seen in liver. Copious haemorrhage. External wound closed. Gradual improvement over four weeks. Patient recovered.

Cases 78 and 79: Wounds of stomach – usually fatal. Preceded by a discussion of treatment.

Case 78 (reported by M. Hevin, France): Two cases of recovery following incised wounds of abdominal wall involving stomach, both repaired by suture.

Case 79: Fatal case of a soldier who suffered from repeated and continual vomiting. Post-mortem showed stomach to resemble tripe, which on section appeared to be honeycombed. ? Pathology.

Followed by discussion by American and French surgeons of fistulous openings into stomach and the removal of various swallowed objects.

Wounds of the spleen are discussed; they are usually fatal.

Cases 80–83: Wounds of the kidney – 'though less fatal are scarcely less dangerous'.

Case 80: Fatal case of musket ball injury to kidney and bowel. No post-mortem.

Case 81 (of Dr Hennen): Musket ball wound to kidney; entry wound anterior and ball removed from posterior exit wound. Repeated attacks of haematuria. Patient recovered after seven weeks. A few months later abscess formed at site of posterior wound, which opened and the discharge was 'of a uriniferous odour'. And then suddenly he passed *per urethram* a hard lump, thought to be a stone, but examination showed it to be 'the cloth which had been driven in by the ball'. [Another extraordinary case – the musket ball must have passed down the ureter into the bladder.]

Case 82: Musket ball injury to kidney; entry and exit wounds present, with damage to fourth and fifth lumbar vertebrae. Urine emerged from posterior wound. Paralysis of one leg and partial paralysis of the other.

The following passage graphically describes the fate of many soldiers during the Peninsular campaign and is worthy of inclusion. The injured man was French, but Guthrie treated enemy soldiers and his own injured soldiers with equal consideration:

> He was left on the field of battle, supposed to be about to die and was brought to me *[Guthrie]* to the village of Valverde three days afterwards in the most distressing state. The inflammatory symptoms were subdued but his condition, from want of almost every comfort after the bloodiest battle in British history *[Albuhera]* was to be deplored. The pain he suffered on any attempt to move him was excessive, the discharge of faeces from the anterior

wound and of urine from the posterior one, and by the usual ways, rendered him miserable, and he at last implored me to allow him the box of opium pills, of which one was given at night to each man who stood most in need of them, to be left within his reach, if I would not kindly do the act of a friend and give them to him myself. He died at the end of ten days after great suffering, constantly regretting that our feelings as Christians caused their prolongation.

Case 83: Fatal case of injury to kidney and colon.

Cases 84–87: Wounds of the spermatic cord 'rarely lead to fatal, though often inconvenient, consequences'; e.g. an injury to both corpora cavernosa in a married soldier – 'the man suffered very little inconvenience ... he seemed to consider the injury of no importance to himself but had some idea there might be a difference of opinion in another party'.

Lecture 6

Wounds of the pelvis from musket balls, injuring its contents, are of common occurrence and although frequently fatal, they are not usually so at the moment, and often permit of a considerable length of treatment before they destroy the sufferers or admit of their recovery. In a great number the ingenuity of the surgeon is often at work to discover in what manner important, nay vital, parts have escaped injury.

Cases 88–111: Wounds of the pelvis treated by Guthrie, other English surgeons, Barons Larrey and Percy, Dupuytren, Langenbech and others are described, but are too complicated to summarize.

Reference

1. *Lancet* 1853; **1**: 399–401.

CHAPTER 22

Wounds and Injuries of the Chest *(1848)*

W*ounds and Injuries of the Chest* (Figure 22.1) was published in 1848 and was the first English book devoted entirely to chest injuries and diseases. Much of its content had been included in Guthrie's major work *Commentaries on the Surgery of the War*, first published in 1815, and it shows that Guthrie had considerable insight into the rational treatment of chest trauma and disease. The 109 pages record 13 lectures and include 164 detailed case histories of patients who had sustained chest wounds. The fatal cases include the post-mortem findings. Except where stated otherwise the injuries were all treated by Guthrie; many of the French patients were treated by Baudens, Dupuytren, Larrey and Percy.

These lectures on the chest were printed in *The Lancet* in 1853 as Lectures 10–17 in a series of *Some of the More Important Points in Surgery*.[1]

Guthrie must have had a special interest in thoracic surgery although, of course, chest injuries would have occupied a considerable part of his work in the Peninsular War. He was

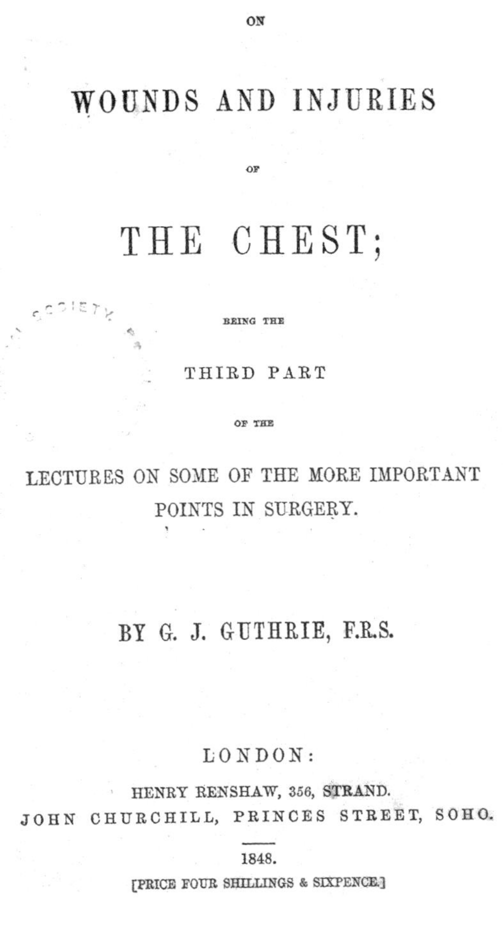

Figure 22.1 *Title page of* Wounds and Injuries of the Chest, *published in 1848 (reproduced with permission from the Royal College of Surgeons of England)*

ON

WOUNDS AND INJURIES

OF

THE CHEST;

BEING THE

THIRD PART

OF THE

LECTURES ON SOME OF THE MORE IMPORTANT
POINTS IN SURGERY.

BY G. J. GUTHRIE, F.R.S.

LONDON:

HENRY RENSHAW, 356, STRAND.
JOHN CHURCHILL, PRINCES STREET, SOHO.

1848.

[PRICE FOUR SHILLINGS & SIXPENCE.]

responsible for many important advances in the treatment of these injuries and these are enumerated in some detail in Chapter 8.

In the Introductory Lecture to *Wounds and Injuries of the Arteries* published in 1830 Guthrie had complained that:

> Many of the gentlemen who come before me at the Court of Examiners of the College of Surgeons are exceedingly ill-informed on the subject of chest injuries. Some do not even know, when a man is stabbed on the right side of the chest, whether he should lie on that side, on the other side, or on his back, and, even if they should answer correctly, it is by no means uncommon for them not to be able to give a reason for the selection. I can safely say that scarcely one student that I have examined in the eighteen years I have been an examiner has been able to tell me the proper treatment to be pursued with regard to an incised wound of the chest.

Even the members of Council considered that a chest wound should be allowed to remain open and that venesection and enemata were the preferred treatments.

Preface

Most of the Preface is devoted to outspoken criticism of the administration of the army medical services throughout the Peninsular campaign and for a considerable time afterwards.

The casualties from four battles in India had been returned to England and when they arrived at Chatham Guthrie found to his dismay that only seven had suffered chest injuries. The casualties in these four battles had been three times those at Toulouse and 'by computation the proportionate number of men shot through the chest and sent to England should have been 171 instead of 7' (another instance of the value of statistics, introduced into the army by Guthrie – see Chapter 8, p. 130). He had complained to the government and asked why this situation had arisen but, at the time of writing this Preface two years later, he had had no response. 'The cause is well known – the remedy in great part attainable. The evil remains', his Preface concludes.

Finally, he criticized the army administration and wrote what could also be said about the recent Afghanistan conflict:

> The Royal Army of Great Britain is not composed of mercenaries. Its soldiers are the blood, the bone, the sinew of the

nation, on whose indomitable valour alone can dependence be placed in the hour of danger. By them the victory must be won, by them the loss must be sustained; and a country grateful for their services should watch over them in their necessities, as a mother over her children.

General conclusions for the treatment of chest injuries ('subject to certain deviations')

These are described in Chapter 8, page 133.

Summary of the book

The book contributes much more than its title would suggest, for lectures 1–7 (of 13 lectures) deal entirely with medical, as opposed to surgical, conditions – the natural history of pneumonia and emphysema, together with their diagnosis by auscultation and percussion and the significance of pectoriloquy ('chest talking'). Throughout the lectures the importance of the use of the stethoscope is emphasized (especially in cases 28, 59, 66 and 69) and numerous cases histories are included, together with post-mortem findings if applicable. The first three lectures are devoted to diagnosis and to inflammatory conditions of the lung.

Especially interesting or unusual cases are cases 21 and 24 (expectorated empyema), case 28 (value of stethoscope), case 35 (treatment of surgical emphysema), case 52 (recovery from heart injury), case 58 (empyema drainage by making patient speak), case 61 (fencing accident in which foil passed through both sides of chest), case 69 (treatment of haemothorax), case 74 (importance of *dependent* drainage of empyema), case 81 (penetrating chest wound), case 109 (very large shot wound), cases 136 and 137 (unusual techniques for empyema drainage – one successful and one not), case 139 (empyema drainage), case 147 (strangulated diaphragmatic hernia), cases 154 and 155 (transfixion injuries of chest) and case 162 (silver mask to cover severe loss of lower jaw).

Venesection was advised in many of these case reports, as had been advised in previous centuries, and Guthrie considered that this prevented the onset of pneumonia. Venesection continued to be advised as late as 1896 when Paget said in his book, *Surgery of the Chest*, that 'there is abundant evidence that venesection may bring immediate relief or may even, as far as we can judge, save the patient's life'.[2] There was, in fact, some merit in this procedure before the introduction of blood transfusion in that the lowered blood pressure would encourage clotting of the blood and so arrest the haemorrhage. Patients were frequently bled until they fainted from loss of blood. The temporal artery was sometimes used if no blood could be obtained from an arm vein (see Lecture 10, cases 82–88 and Lecture 11). Perhaps, surprisingly, the venesection quite frequently relieved the symptoms of 'oppression of the chest' or difficulty in breathing.

Lecture 1: General remarks concerning chest injuries

A knowledge of physic is inseparable from the practise of surgery; it is especially so in the treatment of injuries of the chest' *[i.e. medical knowledge – how true of modern cardiothoracic surgery, and one of the reasons why the author found this specialty so fascinating]* .... The practice of surgery ought never to be separated from the practice of physic if the surgeon is to take sole charge of accidents. If the surgeon is to be any other than the mere drudge or artist he must first learn the principles and he must then continually engage in the practice of physic.

The value of the newly discovered art of auscultation is stressed and the different types of respiration and their significance are described – vesicular breathing, pectoriloquy ('chest talking') and broncophony. This is followed by a discussion of incised wounds by bayonet or knife, which must be managed differently from blunt injury by musket ball. Ten cases of blunt injury are described and their treatment discussed; complications were haemoptysis, pneumonia and, in one case, gangrene of the lung. The stethoscope was thought to be more valuable than percussion, which often caused considerable pain after a chest injury.

Cases 1–9: Blunt non-penetrating injuries to chest wall. Complications were haemoptysis and pneumonia.

Case 10: (of Dr Stokes, Dublin): Blunt injury, followed by pneumonia and lung abscess. Patient died. Post-mortem. An extended discussion of diagnosis of a lung abscess by auscultation follows.

An interesting remark concerning bayonet wounds is included. Though regiments advance with fixed bayonets and intend to engage their foe, quite often valour gives way to discretion and the combatants walk 'silently and angrily' away. Many bayonet injuries resulted in rapid death and few were seen by a surgeon.

Lecture 2: Inflammation of the pleura and of the lung

Inflammation of the pleura, leading to effusion and in some cases empyema, together with the three stages of pneumonia, are discussed. A discussion follows of the changing physical signs during these three stages, their significance and their relationship to the prognosis. Persisting pleural effusion after pneumonia frequently leads to 'false membrane' formation (fibrin and therefore thickened pleura) in the chest.

Lecture 3: The histological changes in pneumonia

The three stages of pneumonia, first described by Laennec and investigated by Andral, are: (1) *engorgement* (12 hours to 3 days); (2) the *hepatization* of Laennec and *red softening* of Andral (1–3 days); and (3) *purulent infiltration* of both. These are all described in detail, together with the opinions of Stokes (Dublin) and of French physicians.

The value of *venesection* is discussed in considerable detail. Guthrie himself was a great advocate of this treatment, though he accepted that it was very controversial, especially amongst French physicians. In the young, 'bleeding should be repeated until the object is effected', i.e. relief of pain and difficulty in breathing.

> The quantity required to be drawn in inflammation, particularly after injuries, is often very great. It is almost a question, in some cases, whether the patient shall be allowed to die of the disease or from loss of blood.

It should be done, he said, 'in a very determined manner' and repeated every four hours in the first stage until the patient fainted, though he agreed it was less effective in the second stage (see also case 85 and Lecture 11). Oral tartar emetic was also advised by Guthrie during the first stage and mercury combined with opium in the second stage.

Lecture 4: Typhoid pneumonia and empyema

Typhoid pneumonia and its symptoms are discussed and vene-section was thought inadvisable.

The diagnosis of empyema, a name given by early writers to any abscess in the body and by later writers to a collection of fluid in the chest and also the operation to evacuate it, is discussed, the physical signs described and drainage advised in most cases.

Case 11 (of Dr Golding, England): The treatment of pneumonia in a 17-year-old youth is described.

Lecture 5: The treatment of empyema

The treatment of empyema is discussed in great detail, operation for which is said to have been performed in ancient times by Phalereus, Jason or Prometheus, and it is said of all three that they had been thought to have an incurable 'lung abscess' (i.e. empyema), with such a bad prognosis that each had resolved to die gloriously in battle rather than die ignominiously in bed. Each therefore deliberately advanced towards an advancing enemy; however, they were struck on the chest by a sword, which thus released the pus and cured the empyema.

Drainage by trocar and cannula should be performed 'much more frequently than it is at present' and the site for this is discussed. If an external swelling develops (*empyema necessitas*) it should be incised ('an operation by necessity'), and this was not uncommon after gunshot wounds. Operations by other surgeons (Davies and Roe in England, and Dupuytren and Broussais in France) are reviewed.

The entry of air into the chest is discussed in some detail and Guthrie considered that it did no harm, although others, in particular French surgeons, disagreed and had attached a bladder to the cannula to receive the fluid and prevent the entry of air.

Guthrie summarized his opinion: 'in all cases of serous effusion the fluid should be evacuated and the wound closed. When the fluid is purulent a permanent drain should be early established'.

Cases of empyema treated by Hughes, Thompson and Davies are quoted; Hughes performed puncture 15 times for a serous effusion but, on the other hand, Davies, anticipating the need for several aspirations, inserted a gum-elastic catheter to avoid repeated puncture and provide more continual drainage.

Irrigation was thought to be of questionable value, though it might assist the removal of foreign bodies such as cloth or bone fragments from the pleural cavity.

In this lecture there is some confusion as to when serous or purulent effusions are being discussed. But it must be remembered that the book was written in 1848, a few years before Lister's momentous paper in 1867 in which the cause and prevention of infection were established.

Case 12 (of Dr Goza, Marseilles): Case of pneumonia followed by a large effusion, drained by trocar and cannula.

Case 13 (of Dr Morand, England): Empyema drained for nine months – sinus healed, recovery.

Case 14 (of Dr Diemerbrock): Successful drainage of empyema.

Case 15 (of Dr Wendalstadt, Hersfield): Flattened and contracted chest wall due to a chronic drained empyema. After 13 years rib sequestrum removed – ? final outcome.

Case 16: GSW (gunshot wound) chest – drainage not dependent; redrainage advised but refused, and patient died later.

Case 17: GSW chest – open wound healed but empyema remained; immediate improvement after redrainage. Patient recovered.

Case 18: GSW chest – chronic empyema drained but patient died. Grossly thickened pleura at post-mortem.

Case 19: GSW chest – empyema drained, with release of rib fragments and pieces of cloth; relapse later and patient died. No post-mortem.

Case 20: Post-mortem appearances in a patient with a chronic empyema of three years' duration.

Case 21 (of Mr Lynn, Westminster Hospital): GSW chest, empyema drained; redrainage; bronchopleural fistula developed, patient died, post-mortem (Figure 22.2).

Lecture 6: Empyema and pneumothorax

Cases 22 and 23: Acute empyema, drainage; patient died, post-mortem.

Case 24: Empyema and bronchopleural fistula. Complete recovery after expectoration of four pints of pus.

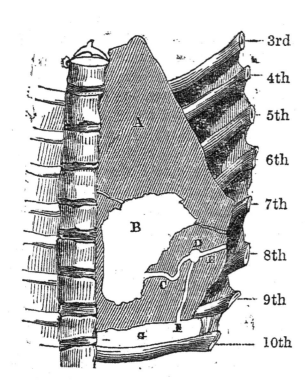

3rd
4th
5th
6th
7th
8th
9th
10th

Figure 22.2 *Bronchopleural fistula. A, section of lung made vertically; B, abscess, communicating through a sinus C with a cavity D, in which the ball had lodged through a sinus E. The ball had passed into the chest between the seventh and eighth ribs, to which the lung was adherent*

Pneumothorax and its diagnosis is then discussed, divided into spontaneous pneumothorax ('beginning of a disease') and pneumothorax complicating tuberculosis ('end of a disease').

Case 25: Spontaneous pneumothorax relieved by trocar and cannula.

Cases 26 and 27 (of Dr Johnson and Dr Bird): Pneumothorax due to tuberculosis. Post-mortem.

Case 28: GSW below right nipple 'when standing sideways'. Over next three hours increasing dyspnoea relieved by four-pint venesection 'until pulse failed' and this relieved the dyspnoea – over next week daily recurrence of dyspnoea relieved each time by application of leeches to chest, to a total of 265 leeches. Gradual improvement until a month later when dyspnoea returned – signs of a left pneumothorax appeared. Gum-elastic catheter introduced through GSW into left chest led to instant relief, catheter introduced daily for next week. Patient recovered. [This case is reported at length to show the type of treatment in 1832 and what 'strict and constant watching such cases require'; 'unremitting use of the stethoscope', he writes in case 69).

Lecture 7: Surgical emphysema, hernia of the lung and heart wounds

Cases 29–32: Cases of surgical emphysema following chest injury previously reported by Paré, Wiseman, Littre and W. Hunter.

Emphysema of lung: Brief description of this medical condition.

Surgical emphysema (subcutaneous air following a wound of the lung) described following fractured ribs – treatment by compression bandage advised, following which two patients (cases 33 and 34) treated by Larrey are included.

Case 35: Sword wound leading to surgical emphysema and treated by enlargement of wound to release the air, followed by compression bandage. Differing opinions on the treatment of surgical emphysema are discussed.

Cases 36 and 37 (of M. Sabatier and M. Voisin, Limoges): Discussion of treatment of hernia of the lung.

Cases 38–41 (of Drs Babington, Featherstone, Davis and Trigger, England): Wounds of the heart are not always immediately fatal and many previous reports of survival for a few hours or days are described. Three such recent cases treated by Guthrie are included.

Lecture 8: Wounds of the heart

Cases 42–51: Short-term survival of heart wounds reported by Dupuytren, Percy, Velpau and others are described, together with four long-term survivors.

Surface markings of the heart and its contents are described. *Heart sounds and murmurs* are analysed. *Wounds of the pericardium* (four cases) reported by Larrey in his *Memoires* are included. *Drainage of the pericardium* – subcostal technique by Larrey and trephination of sternum by Skielderup, are both described in detail.

Case 52: Detailed description of post-mortem findings in a battle of Waterloo casualty who had recovered from a lance injury which had penetrated the anterior chest wall one year previously. Death had occurred from unrelated pneumonia. The lance had passed through the left lower lobe of lung, 'sliced a piece of the right ventricle', passed through the diaphragm and entered the liver (Figure 22.3).

Case 53: Needles in the heart reported by a Russian surgeon and by Hennen are briefly included. Both patients died.

Case 54 (of Dr O'Connor): Successful removal of a darning needle from the heart.

Figure 22.3 *Heart wound. A and B, right and left ventricle; C and D, right and left atrium; E, F and G, aorta, pulmonary and coronary artery; H, rib cartilage; I, diaphragm; K, pericardium; 1, portion of pericardium; 2, opening of wound in diaphragm and pericardium; 3, pendulous slice of substance of right ventricle; 4, puckered cicatrix of wound of ventricle*

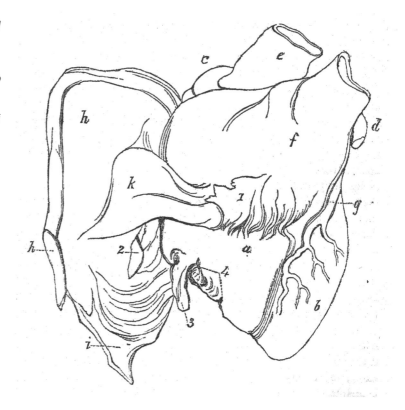

Lecture 9: Penetrating wounds of the chest

This important lecture is devoted to the treatment of penetrating wounds of the chest. Twenty-one case histories (cases 55–76, some treated in the 17th and 18th centuries, some treated by Guthrie, and two cases treated by Larrey) are described and all are interspersed with Guthrie's own opinions and criticisms of their treatment. He accepts that the treatment of these wounds is controversial (for his 'general conclusions' for the treatment of penetrating chest wounds see Chapter 8, p. 133).

Early closure of chest wounds, first advised in the 14th century but soon forgotten, was repeatedly recognized in the following centuries but not finally accepted until World War I, 600 years later.[3] In the early 19th century Guthrie was adamant that open chest wounds should be closed as soon as possible (see case 69).

Simple incised wounds should always be closed after making sure 'that no portion of the offending instrument is broken off and sticking in'. Guthrie stressed the danger of probing a chest wound.

Case 55 (of Dr Mayer): Knife wound – broken blade not removed for several days. Infection occurred and recovery was therefore delayed. Discussion of views of Paré, Würtz and La Motte in similar cases.

Cases 56–58 (of La Motte in the 17th century): Sword wounds causing haemothorax without damage to the lung. The use of human 'suckers' (originated by French surgeon Anel) to remove blood from the pleural cavity is mentioned; Anel subsequently devised a more hygienic suction apparatus to withdraw blood from the pleural cavity (case 58).[3] Patient advised to lie on injured side to allow the lung to be closely applied to the chest wall, in the hope that adhesions would cut off the wound from the general thoracic cavity.

Case 59: Bayonet wound. 'Auscultation should always be resorted to from the moment of injury and constantly used throughout the treatment'.

Case 60: Multiple bayonet wounds. Patient died.

Case 61 (of Mr Keate): Fencing accident – the foil passed through the chest from right to left and out the other side. Patient recovered.

Case 62: Penetrating wound from musket ball – paradoxical respiration. Patient died.

Cases 63 and 64: Penetrating sword wounds – sutured. Patients recovered.

Case 65 (of Mr Stanley): Knife wound (anterior), with posterior exit wound. Patient recovered. ? Treatment.

Case 66 (of Dr Foltz, American Navy): Knife wound sutured – haemothorax evacuated five days later. Patient recovered. 'From the moment the wound is closed the stethoscope and the ear become the most important guides.'

Cases 67 and 68: Sword wound – late evacuation of haemo-thorax. Both patients died.

Case 69: Sabre wound.

Extensive discussion follows on the closure of open chest wounds and the controversial treatment of haemothorax. An open chest wound must always be closed 'to relieve the breathing'. Guthrie quotes a report in *The Lancet* of an open chest causing paradoxical respiration – the air had 'issued from the wound at each respiration with a whizzing noise – the wound was kept open and the patient died next day, *in all probability from its having been so done'.*[4] Concerning the treatment of haemorrhage into the chest, Guthrie advised removal of as much blood as possible ('evacuated by position') before closure of the wound. He wrote:

> As the bleeding vessel in the lung cannot readily be got at if seen, and if got at cannot be secured by ligature, the only means left, if the bleeding continue, is to close the wound and allow the cavity of the pleura to be filled, until the lung be sufficiently compressed to cause the haemorrhage to cease, if the patient should survive so long.

The closure of the wound might be sufficient to arrest the haemorrhage. 'The first object is to save life', he said, 'after that, if time be given, the next will be to relieve the loaded cavity, but what time will be required to render the suppression of the bleeding permanent has not yet been clearly ascertained'. Larrey advised reopening the chest to evacuate the blood after 10 days. Guthrie 'ventured to disagree' and considered five days only should elapse:

> The probability of a return of the bleeding is not great after an early opening has been made, although much mischief will inevitably follow the effused fluids remaining too long; the blood should be removed lest infection occur. ... To ascertain the proper time for doing this when the wound is not open requires great care and unremitting attention in the use of the stethoscope.

Case 70: Sword wounds in the 18th century. The views of Pierre Dionis (Paris) in 1710 and of Le Dran (Paris) in 1740 concerning open chest wounds were identical to those of Guthrie – *they should always be closed.*

Cases 71 and 72: Sword wounds – late evacuation of haemothorax. Both patients recovered.

Case 73: Sword wounds. The policy of Valentin (France) in 1772 of early closure of a penetrating wound and later evacuation of a haemothorax did not receive the credit due to him. 'The recommendations of Larrey and those of others as well as my own add nothing to what he had already said; they have only enforced what had been neglected'. (Surprisingly this vital policy[3] was repeatedly forgotten even up to World War I.)

Case 74 (of Pechlin in the 18th century): Sword wound – haemothorax. Repeated introduction and withdrawal of a bougie to evacuate the blood, empyema (unsurprising because of inevitable introduction of infection in pre-Listerian days). Patient recovered. In the previous century Valentin had commented on a similar injury and said: 'if instead of keeping the wound open by a tent they had allowed it to close and had made a counter-opening at the place of election when the symptoms of effusion had appeared to require it, the patient would have escaped with much less suffering'. Valentin had also commented on the occurrence of *ecchymosis* over the lower chest and descending towards the loins; this would appear about 10 days after the injury and was considered to be pathognomonic of a haemothorax.

Case 75 (of Larrey): Sword wound – recovery after 10 months. Larrey's treatment of this patient was criticized by Guthrie.

Case 76 (of Larrey): Sword wound – ecchymosis noted three days after injury. Larrey revived the views of Valentin so effectively that they were attributed to Larrey himself; in fact they had been noted previously by La Motte and by Ravaton.

Lecture 10: Musket ball injuries

In many musket ball injuries there was an associated rib fracture, and fragments of bone, together with buttons and pieces of clothing, were subsequently removed. These case histories provide considerable insight into how battles were fought in the early 19th century, how the injured were removed from the scene of battle and how they were managed. Many of the casualties were high-ranking officers who had led from the front.

The entry wound was usually 'round, depressed, dark coloured and bloody' whilst the exit wound was 'more of a rugged slit or tear than a hole'. Guthrie considered wounds in the upper chest to be more dangerous than those in the lower chest.

The ball only rarely remained in the lung – it usually passed right through the chest or lodged in the chest wall near the entry or exit wound within the intercostal space. In some cases the ball ran around the inner chest wall after entering the chest.

Most of these cases of musket ball injury recovered and many returned to duty.

Cases 77 and 78 (of Ravaton and Guthrie): Entry wound in anterior chest wall.

Case 79: Ball lodged in intercostal space. Discussion follows on debridement of the wound. If the wound is enlarged this 'should be no greater in extent than is absolutely necessary for the purpose intended'.

Case 80: Further discussion of debridement – spicules of bone to be removed and ends of rib rounded off. If the ball hits a rib cartilage it usually passes through it and bends it; this can easily be corrected.

Case 81: Musket ball injury to chest and abdomen. Ball entered anterior chest, ran round inner side of the ribs and emerged near angle of the rib. Patient died from peritonitis due to an abdominal wound.

Cases 82–88: Penetrating musket ball injuries – with an entry and exit wound. All patients recovered. Case 85 was bled from the temporal artery each time until the haemorrhage ceased.

Cases 89 and 90: Penetrating musket ball injuries.

Case 91 (of M. Scharf, Germany): Gored by a bull – rib fractures and haemothorax. Patient recovered.

Cases 92–107: Musket ball injuries. Cases 96–105 describe injuries associated with 'formation of matter and ultimate recovery' (i.e. infection), but with later chest deformity.

Cases 108 and 109: Two cases of injury by large shot. In case 109 the shot weighed two pounds and passed right through the chest, causing a wound so large that his commanding officer could 'see the light quite through him'. Both patients recovered.

Lecture 11: Penetrating chest injuries from musket balls

This is a somewhat tedious lecture to read. Twenty-five detailed case histories of penetrating musket ball injury of the chest are described, many treated by Guthrie and others by Home and Key (London) and Larrey, Guérin and Percy (France). One soldier had been left on the battlefield for four days (not infrequent in the 19th century) and many of the injured had retained clothing, buttons or leather in the chest. Only six of these soldiers recovered from their wounds. In one case the temporal artery had been bled, 'as no blood could be drawn from the veins'. Case 124 is followed by a discussion on retained foreign material after musket ball injury – the patient rarely survived unless this was removed.

Lecture 12: Musket ball injuries and wounds of the diaphragm

A preliminary paragraph summarizes the effect of a penetrating chest wound. An early effusion often develops, becomes infected and leads to thickening of the pleura, which may become one inch thick. 'Nature makes some efforts, which are usually unavailing, to relieve herself by an external opening'. If the patient survives long enough, an *empyema necessitas* will develop and discharge spontaneously. If the empyema is drained in these cases the lung 'can rarely again expand', leading to elevation of the diaphragm, shift of the mediastinum and a flattened deformed chest wall. 'Under such circumstances it must be obvious that these evils can only be prevented by an early operation, capable of giving a ready exit to the matter secreted and to any foreign substance which may have fallen into the cavity of the chest' (an accurate summary of opinion concerning empyema after penetrating injury until as late as 1950).

Case 134 (of Gérard, France): Bilateral musket ball injury of the chest, one ball having penetrated the diaphragm. Recovery after extraction of ball from abdomen.

Case 135 (of Dupuytren, France): Pistol ball injury of chest – fatal outcome. Guthrie commented that auscultation had not been utilized and that 'no effective means were taken for the relief of the patient, save bleeding'. The use of Anel's (France) suction pump is discussed[3] (see Lecture 9, case 58), which later was also advised by Sabatier.

Case 136 (of Baudens, France): Musket ball injury to upper chest. A bougie was introduced and 'made to project between the eleventh and twelfth ribs'. The ball and several rib splinters were removed through an incision over this. The lower wound was closed, the upper wound sucked daily by pump and the patient recovered in 40 days. The operation was described by Guthrie as 'a very brilliant result of modern surgery'.

Case 137 (of Baudens, France): Empyema following musket ball injury treated by daily aspiration of pus for five days, followed by closure of the wound. Patient died eight days later. Guthrie correctly commented that dependent drainage was obligatory and that 'if instead of pumping out the chest the posterior wound had been re-opened the sufferer might, I apprehend, have had a better chance'.

Case 138 (of Baudens, France): Empyema following musket ball injury – inadequate drainage and patient died. Guthrie agreed with Bauden's own criticism of the treatment of this case.

Case 139 (of Baudens, France): Similar to case 138. Guthrie emphasizes the danger of draining an empyema too low and therefore opening the abdomen by mistake, an error very easily made. [This error was made by the author when he was a junior surgical registrar in 1946. The wound was closed, the empyema drained higher up and the patient recovered uneventfully.] He then describes at length a series of dissections which he had undertaken at the Royal College of Surgeons and at Charing Cross Hospital to show how this error could be avoided.

Wounds of the diaphragm are discussed next, following earlier case reports of such cases by Paré, Sennerus, Hollerius, Guillemeau and Chevreau.

Cases 140–148: Case reports of injury to the diaphragm, most of which were only diagnosed at post-mortem and several of which were associated with herniation of the stomach or colon into the chest. Cases reported by Dupuytren and Percy (both French) are also included. Case 147 reports a soldier who recovered from a sword wound of the diaphragm and who developed symptoms of an 'internal rupture' 15 months later whilst cleaning his horse. He died the next day and post-mortem examination showed a strangulated stomach inside the chest.

Cases 149–152: Two case reports by Guthrie, one by Larrey and one by Baudens, of penetrating chest wound associated with diaphragmatic injury.

Finally, Guthrie states that he was the first to point out that wounds of the muscular and tendinous part of the diaphragm never unite and therefore such injuries may later be associated with a diaphragmatic hernia.

Lecture 13: Herniation of the lung, internal mammary and intercostal artery wounds, and wounds of the head and neck

A hernia (protrusion) of the lung through a chest wound should not be replaced inside the chest but should be allowed to remain outside the chest and become adherent to the pleura. Historical cases described by Roland in 1264, Tulpius, Hildanus and Raysch are briefly described. Guthrie then describes three cases successfully treated at the battle of Waterloo. Another case treated at Waterloo by Mr S. Cooper by ligature and excision did not survive.

Case 153 (of D'Anglois, France): Lung hernia after chest wound in a child. Patient recovered.

Case 154 (of Mr Andrews, London Hospital): Transfixion of chest close to sternum by an iron bolt. Patient recovered.

Case 155: Transfixion of chest by shaft of a gig (Mr Tipple's celebrated chest wound). The shaft passed left to right *behind* the sternum. The patient survived (for further details of this extraordinary case see references 5–7). The treatment of internal mammary artery injuries, though rare, is discussed, as also is that of an intercostal artery injury.

Case 156: Larrey's case of possible internal mammary artery injury.

Cases 157–160: Intercostal artery injury treated by local pressure (case 158 of Mr S. Cooper led to a very large infected haematoma).

There is a short section on *wounds of the head and neck* which begins with some general remarks.

Case 161 (of M. Breschet, Paris): Musket ball injury to side of neck – secondary haemorrhage a few days later. Ligation of common carotid artery proposed by Breschet (Paris) but patient died before the operation was performed. Guthrie warns against such an operation. Post-mortem showed that the *vertebral* artery had been damaged, not the carotid.

Case 162 (of M. Paillard and Marx, Antwerp): Loss of lower jaw caused by shell fragment in 1832. The use of a silver mask to cover the lower jaw injury is described.

Case 163: Pistol ball injury involving upper jaw.

Case 164: Musket ball injury involving lower jaw.

References

1. Some of the More Important Points in Surgery. *Lancet* 1853; **1**: 217–9 (Lecture 10 on pleuritis and pneumonia), 239–40 and 261–4 (Lecture 11 on empyema), 285–8 (Lecture 12 on emphysema), 309–12 (Lecture 13 on gunshot wounds of the chest), 331–4 (Lecture 14 on the post-mortem appearances after chest injury), 355–9 (Lecture 15 on lung hernia, wounds of diaphragm and head), 377–9 (Lecture 16 on wounds of internal mammary and intercostal arteries, wounds of neck and eye), 399–401 (Lecture 17 on abdominal wounds) (issues of 5 March–30 April).
2. Paget S. *Surgery of the Chest*. Bristol: Wright, 1896, p. 325.
3. Hurt R. *History of Cardiothoracic Surgery from Early Times*. London: Parthenon, 1996, pp. 237–9, 249.
4. Case of a wound penetrating the cavity of the thorax (no named author). *Lancet* 1825; **8**: 94–5.
5. Wood S. Mr Tipple's chest wound. *Ann R Coll Surg Engl* 1961; **28**: 122–30.
6. Earle P. Case of Thomas Tipple. *Am J Med Sci* 1841; **2**: 117–21.
7. Op. cit. ref. 2, p. 262.

Index of Names

Index

Page references to **figures** are shown in **bold**.